Migraine and Other Headaches

WILLIAM B. YOUNG, MD
STEPHEN D. SILBERSTEIN, MD

Jefferson Headache Center
Thomas Jefferson University Hospital
Philadelphia, Pennsylvania

AUSTIN J. SUMNER, MD
Series Editor

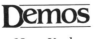

New York

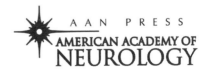

AAN PRESS
AMERICAN ACADEMY OF
NEUROLOGY

Demos Medical Publishing Inc., 368 Park Avenue South, New York, New York 10016

Uses for products within this text may include those not currently approved by the FDA. For more information on the products, please see full prescribing information.

Library of Congress Cataloging-in-Publication Data

Young, William B.
 Migraine and other headaches / by William B. Young and Stephen D. Silberstein. — 1st ed.
  p. ; cm.
 Includes index.
 ISBN 1-932603-03-4 (pbk. : alk. paper)
 1. Migraine. 2. Headache.
 [DNLM: 1. Migraine. 2. Headache Disorders. WL 344 S582m 2004] I. Silberstein, Stephen D. II. Title.
 RC392.S524 2004
 616.8'491—dc22

                                                    2004000976

Printed in Canada

Contents

SECTION I
HISTORY, PHILOSOPHY, AND GENERAL CONCEPTS

CHAPTER 1

CHAPTER 2

CHAPTER 3

CHAPTER 4

Contents

SECTION II
PRIMARY HEADACHE—MIGRAINE

SECTION III
OTHER PRIMARY HEADACHES AND ASSOCIATED ILLNESSES

SECTION IV
SECONDARY HEADACHE

About the AAN Press Quality of Life Guides

IN THE SPIRIT OF THE DOCTOR-PATIENT PARTNERSHIP

THE BETTER-INFORMED PATIENT is often able to play a vital role in his or her own care. This is especially the case with neurologic disorders, for which effective management of disease can be promoted—indeed, *enhanced*—through patient education and involvement.

In the spirit of the partnership-in-care between physicians and patients, the American Academy of Neurology Press is pleased to produce a series of "Quality of Life" guides on an array of diseases and ailments that affect the brain and central nervous system. The series, produced in partnership with Demos Medical Publishing, answers a number of basic and important questions faced by patients and their families.

Additionally, the authors, most of whom are physicians and all of whom are experts in the areas in which they write, provide a detailed discussion of the disorder, its causes, and the course it may follow. You also find strategies for coping with the disorder and handling a number of nonmedical issues.

The result: as a reader, you will be able to develop a framework for understanding the disease and become better prepared to manage the life changes associated with it.

ABOUT THE AMERICAN ACADEMY OF NEUROLOGY (AAN)

The American Academy of Neurology is the premier organization for neurologists worldwide. In addition to support of educational and scientific advances, the AAN—along with its sister organization, the AAN Foundation – is a strong advocate of public education and a leading supporter of research for breakthroughs in neurologic patient care.

More information on the activities of the AAN is available on our website, www.aan.com. For a better understanding of common disorders of the brain, as well as to learn about people living with these disorders, please turn to the AAN Foundation's website, www.thebrainmatters.org.

ABOUT NEUROLOGY AND NEUROLOGISTS

Neurology is the medical specialty associated with disorders of the brain and central nervous system. Neurologists are medical doctors with specialized training in the diagnosis, treatment, and management of patients suffering from neurologic disease.

Austin J. Sumner, M.D.
Series Editor, AAN Press Quality of Life Guides

Foreword

M OST OF US HAVE OCCASIONAL HEADACHES that are relieved by over-the-counter (OTC) medications. When headaches are frequent, severe, or unrelieved by the OTCs, we usually consult our primary care physician (PCPs). Headache is the seventh most common reason for PCP visits, and the most frequent cause of severe recurrent headaches is migraine. Unfortunately, about half of all patients with migraine are not properly diagnosed, and those who are properly diagnosed often don't receive appropriate treatment.

The obvious answer is to educate primary care physicians on the diagnosis and management of migraine. However, despite the two major headache societies in the United States—the American Headache Society and the National Headache Foundation, each providing twice yearly continuing medical education courses aimed at PCPs, we haven't witnessed a major impact on diagnostic accuracy.

Another strategy is patient education. If attempts to educate PCPs are unsuccessful, we can provide information for migraine and other headache sufferers to self-diagnose and provide their doctors with the proper diagnosis, and perhaps even an intelligent approach to treatment. Although there are thousands of Internet sites for headache, they are of variable quality.[1] The same holds for self-help books, but a book sponsored by the American Academy of Neurology is assuredly authoritative. Consider a patient visiting her/his doctor, pointing to the 2004 *International Headache Society Classification*, and saying, "I have '*migraine*' because my recurrent headaches have at least two out of these four, and one out of these two, criteria."

The authors of this book, Drs. Stephen Silberstein and William Young, are distinguished, highly regarded headache specialists. Both are active in the American Academy of Neurology and the American Headache Society (Dr. Silberstein will be assuming the presidency of the latter in 2004).

In addition to uncovering the road to headache relief for current suf-ferers, it will aid patients who are satisfied with their treatment but want to know more about the underlying migraine mechanisms. The authors explain complex concepts simply, without oversimplification.

The early chapters are general, and provide a historical perspective. These are followed by explanations of the causes of head pain in gener-al, those headaches that require urgent medical attention, and advice in finding the "right" headache doctor. Readers are told when to switch doctors (one reason should be a doctor ordering an electroencephalo-gram for monosymptomatic headache), and what historical information they should provide the headache specialist at their first encounter.

The standard treatments are presented with explanations of their mechanisms of action. A chapter on "alternative therapies" lists the available evidence for most such treatments, and the potential side effects. This is done dispassionately without bias, pro or con.

In summary, this book is an excellent guide for those experiencing headaches who want better care or more information about their condition.

Robert B. Daroff, M.D.
President, American Headache Society

1. Peroutka, SJ. *Cephalalgia* 2001;21:20–24.

Preface

HEADACHE IS THE MOST COMMON COMPLAINT for which people see neurologists and the seventh most common reason they visit their primary care doctors. Headache is the third most common cause of missed work and it affects every area of a person's life. Many people who suffer from headaches either treat themselves or attempt to ignore their headaches, and less than half of those suffering the serious pain and other symptoms associated with migraine will visit their physician. Headaches have an extraordinary impact and can seriously undermine the quality of life.

Migraine and Other Headaches begins with a general overview, including an interesting history of headache and a discussion of causes. Did you know that Julius Caesar, Napoleon, Thomas Jefferson, Charles Darwin, Sigmund Freud, Vincent van Gogh, Pablo Picasso, and many other famous people suffered from migraine? There has been an attempt to understand and treat headache for thousands of years. The Ebers Papyrus, an ancient Egyptian prescription for headache, dates from about 1200 B.C. It describes migraine, neuralgia, and shooting head pains. In 400 B.C., Hippocrates described both the visual aura that can precede a migraine headache and its relief by vomiting. Galen introduced the term *migraine*, derived from the Greek word *hemicrania*, meaning "half of the head," in approximately 200 A.D.

Different types of headache are thoroughly explained in easy to understand language, beginning with migraine, which is the most common severe headache, occurring in approximately 12 percent of the U.S. population (approximately 28 million people). Migraine can occur at any age. In children, it is more common in boys, but after puberty, it is much more common in girls. Even very young children are suspected of suffering from migraine, although diagnosing them is almost impossible until they learn to speak. In women, it is most common between ages 40 and 45. Men tend to have migraine at a slightly younger age. This means that it often strikes people in their most economically productive years, which is a big part of the effect that migraine has on society.

We have included specific information about the different types of migraine: *migraine without aura* (previously called *common migraine*), *migraine with aura*, and *basilar migraine*. Emphasis is placed on the necessity of early treatment, the importance of understanding the difference between a headache *cause* and a headache *trigger*, and how to avoid common triggers. *Rebound headache*, caused by the overuse of acute medication, is also a topic of special significance that is discussed in detail. In addition to migraine, the book contains a chapter on tension-type headache, the most common primary headache disorder; 80 percent of us will have a tension-type headache at some time in our lives. There are also chapters describing cluster headache, unusual headaches, non-headache illnesses that frequently accompany headache, sinus headache, disorders of the neck, post-traumatic headache, and atypical facial pain and trigeminal neuralgia.

Establishing the headache profile is a critical factor in accurately diagnosing and appropriately treating headache, and anyone who visits a physician with a headache problem will first be thoroughly evaluated in order to determine what type of headache they have. Headache treatment should be a two-way street, with the patient communicating goals and desires about the preferred headache management, the doctor contributing knowledge and values, and the final plan incorporating both perspectives. Above all, the doctor/patient relationship should be a partnership with open communication.

Treatment options for all types of headache are thoroughly discussed, including the treatment of migraine with medications that can be taken daily to help prevent headache, stop headache pain once it has begun, and prevent worsening of headaches. Responses to medication—both prescription and non-prescription—are highly individualized, and the physician will work with the headache sufferer in order to determine the most beneficial medication options. Managing headache pain goes beyond simply popping pills and, therefore, lifestyle issues are considered, including the possibility of depression or other psychological factors, and family relationships. The doctor may recommend changes in diet in order to avoid triggers, exercise, change in sleeping patterns, or relaxation techniques. Also included is information about alternative therapies, such as vitamins and herbal supplements, physical therapy, acupressure, massage, acupuncture, chiropractic care, craniosacral therapy, hydrotherapy, and yoga. Also covered are behavioral treatments, such as stress-management training and psychotherapy.

We hope that *Migraine and Other Headaches* will help those suffering with headaches, and those who care for them, to gain a deeper understanding of what is known about headache and what is *not* known, allowing them to explore diagnosis and treatment with this knowledge in hand. We are at the threshold of an explosion in the understanding, diagnosis, and treatment of migraine and other headaches, and soon more answers *will* be found.

William B. Young, M.D.
Stephen D. Silberstein, M.D., F.A.C.P.

History, Philosophy, and General Concepts

CHAPTER 1

"Just a Headache"

While driving home from work, Kathy Tennenbaum* was slightly distracted by sparkling lights just to the left of her field of vision. When she turned to see what caused them, they moved away. She shook her head as if to shake them loose and for a moment they disappeared, but within seconds, spears of bright light too dramatic to ignore punctured the left side of her vision and a tingling numbness ran up her left arm. She was concerned, but not frightened, until she looked down at the dashboard and could not read it. In the center of her vision was a blurry patch that frightened her. She lived alone and there was no one to call, so she turned left instead of right and headed for the emergency room at her local hospital, tortured by fears of a brain tumor or other unimagined horror. A stabbing pain seared through her left eye as she pulled into the hospital entrance.

"You had a migraine," the neurologist told her, hours later, as she lay, exhausted but finally, mercifully, pain free, on the uncomfortable ER gurney.

"All that from just a headache?" (Figure 1-1)

"JUST A HEADACHE." How often have you heard that phrase? Headache is such a common complaint that it often goes undetected or untreated. Fewer people actually escape headache than suffer from one at least once in their lives. Despite the fact that most people never see a doctor for their headaches, it is the most common complaint for which they see neurologists, and the seventh most common complaint for which they visit their primary care doctors.

The impact of headache should not be minimized. It is the third most common cause of missed work among chronic disorders and it affects

---

*"Kathy Tennenbaum" is not her real name. Throughout, names have been changed to protect individual privacy.

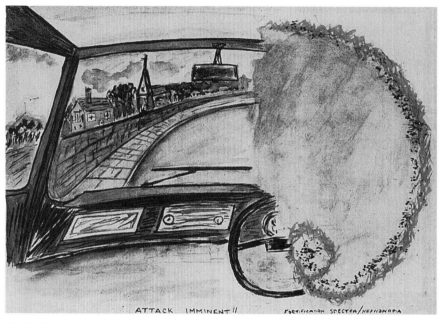

ATTACK IMMINENT !!   FORTIFICATION SPECTRA/HEMIANOPIA

FIGURE 1-1

A sufferer's illustration of the migraine aura.

people at home, at work, in their chores, and in their interactions with friends and family members. It interferes with recreation, exercise, and the pleasures of everyday living. Migraine has an enormous impact on society. In the United States, lost productivity due to migraine costs about 13 billion dollars a year, and four percent of all visits to doctors' offices (over 10 million visits a year) are for headache. Migraine results in major use of emergency rooms and urgent care centers, and vast amounts of prescription and nonprescription medication sales.

Still, most headache sufferers either treat themselves or simply ignore their headaches. Even migraine sufferers tend to put off seeking medical care. Despite the often serious pain and other disturbing symptoms associated with migraine, last year, less than half of those suffering with a headache consulted a doctor for their problem. The reasons for this are many. Widespread misbeliefs about headaches persist. Many people believe that "nothing can really be done," or that it is somehow "weak" to see a doctor for "just a headache" (Figure 1-2).

4

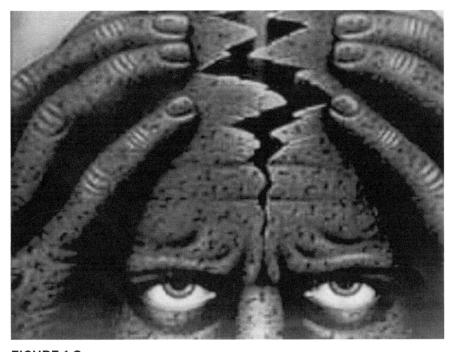

FIGURE 1-2

More than just a headache.

Kathy Tennenbaum was fortunate in many ways. The odds are against a migraine sufferer obtaining speedy relief of symptoms. The visual disturbances that unnerved her served as a warning and, more than the pain that followed, it was these symptoms that led her to seek immediate help at an emergency room. Most people who suffer from migraines do not experience an *aura* (the flashing lights, numbness and tingling, and blurred vision that Kathy experienced). Still, many people, even doctors, believe that without these symptoms, a headache cannot truly be called a migraine. When Kathy described her symptoms to the treating physician, she was referred to a neurologist. She was fortunate in that the neurologist who treated her was knowledgeable about migraine, including the latest treatments, and she was treated appropriately. Once again she was fortunate: she responded well to treatment. Even the newest and most appropriate treatment will not be effective in every case. Kathy Tennenbaum was fortunate, indeed.

Harry Baker was not so fortunate. He thought his head was going to explode. Harry was a tall, heavily built man, attractive, with curly brown hair and hazel eyes, who worked in construction. He was a popular man as well, because he was always ready to do another guy a good turn. That was the only reason he was able to keep his job when he called in sick, again.

"A headache?" his co-worker Bill asked sarcastically when the foreman announced that once again they would be short a man. "Jeez, Lou, we all get headaches!" He rolled his eyes. "This is the second day this week!"

"I don't know, Bill. Louise said he was acting weird, pacing around the house, and he can't sit still. She is trying to get him to go to the doctor, but you know him, he won't go. She says she's worried because one side of his face is all goofy. She thinks he's having a stroke or something."

Harry had undiagnosed cluster headache. Like many of his fellow suffers, he continued to be undiagnosed and untreated until he wound up in a local emergency department. Fortunately for him, the doctor who was on call made the diagnosis and started appropriate treatment.

Headaches can make people miserable. The quality of life of individuals who have chronic, severe headaches is very poor compared with that of people who have other disorders. In general, headache sufferers are worse off than people who have arthritis, roughly similar to those who have congestive heart failure severe enough to interfere with walking up and down stairs, and only slightly better than people with AIDS. Such an extremely poor quality of life is not the reality for all headache

> The quality of life of individuals who have chronic, severe headaches is very poor compared with that of people who have other disorders.

sufferers. However, it does reflect the quality of life of people whose headaches are severe enough for them to seek care at a specialty headache center and the extraordinary impact that headaches can have on an individual's life.

"Be quiet, kids. Your mother has a headache." From her bedroom, Sally Jensen heard her husband Bob's voice in the hall. She had suffered from migraines two or three days every month ever since she reached puberty. Every month, her husband would darken the bedroom where she lay, keep the kids out of trouble and away from her, cook the meals, and run the house. He was a jewel, her friends all told her. She was the luckiest woman on earth. If only she could enjoy it! (Figure 1-3)

Headache, especially migraine, has consequences for friends and family members as well as for the headache sufferer. Migraine is a public health problem of enormous scope. It is the most common severe headache disorder. Twenty-eight million United States residents have severe migraine headaches. Of the people who suffer from severe migraine, 25 percent have four or more attacks a month; 35 percent experience one to four attacks a month; and 40 percent experience less than one attack a month. Most people with severe migraine (82 to 85

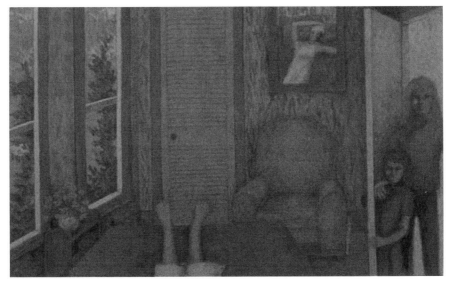

FIGURE 1-3

Serving Time by Nancy Ellen Wheeler; time away from the family.

percent) have some headache-related disability, and about one-third of them are severely disabled or need bed rest. Many migraineurs live in

> Migraine is a public health problem of enormous scope. It is the most common severe headache disorder.

fear between attacks, knowing that at any time an attack can disrupt their ability to work, care for their families, or engage in social activities. Although migraine is often a lifelong disorder, some people experience exacerbations, while others experience remissions, over time.

People who suffer with migraines use about twice as many medical resources—including prescription medicine, office visits, and diagnostic tests—every year as nonmigraineurs. Often the tests that are ordered are not necessary and represent poor understanding on the part of the person who demands the studies or on the part of the doctor who orders them. Expense to society also comes from missed work and from disability. In headache clinics, it is not uncommon to see people who are completely disabled and unable to work because of headaches.

CHAPTER 2

History of Headache

Headache is indelibly linked with the stress and speed of modern life, but it is by no means a modern phenomenon. People have suffered from headaches since the dawn of civilization and, for as long as headaches have existed, so have headache treatments. Well-known migraine suffer-

> People have suffered from headaches since the dawn of civilization and, for as long as headaches have existed, so have headache treatments.

ers—or migraineurs—include Julius Caesar, Napoleon, Ulysses S. Grant, Thomas Jefferson, Robert E. Lee, Charles Darwin, Sigmund Freud, Vincent van Gogh, Pablo Picasso, and Lewis Carroll. A comprehensive list of famous historical headache sufferers—and their sometimes unique treatments—would fill more space than this book allows. What is surprising is that modern medicine still resorts to similar treatments.

Trepanation is a procedure that has been performed since 7000 B.C., in which the skull is perforated with an instrument. Trepanation may have been done to release the demons and evil spirits that were believed to cause headaches, madness, and epilepsy, but it may also have been done for medical reasons. Some African tribes continued to practice trepanation today—without anesthesia—primarily for relief of headache or removal of a fracture line after head injury. Surprisingly, it is also used in Western society. There are still modern trepanation practitioners (see www.trepanation.com) (Figure 2-1).

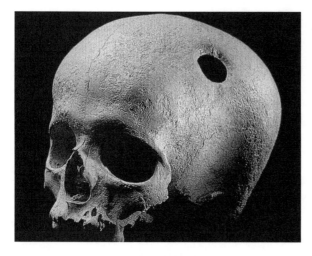

FIGURE 2-1

Trepanation–this patient had a hole drilled in his skull–and survived!

For thousands of years, the medical and popular literature has described headache triggers, relieving factors, and the signs and symptoms of migraine, including headache, aura, nausea and/or vomiting, and familial tendency. References to headache are found as far back as 3000 B.C. The earliest published reference is a Sumerian epic poem, which gives an early description of the *sick headache*:

> The sick-eyed says not
> "I am sick-eyed"
> The sick-headed not
> "I am sick-headed."

This could be interpreted in two ways: headache sufferers 5,000 years ago were either searching for an explanation other than *headache* for what afflicted them, or they preferred to hide their affliction from others. Both these situations are still common today.

The Ebers Papyrus, an ancient Egyptian prescription for headache, dates from about 1200 B.C., and is said to be based on medical documents from 2500 B.C. It describes migraine, neuralgia, and shooting head pains. Like other ancients, the Egyptians believed that the gods could cure their ailments if they followed divine instructions (Figure 2-2A). A clay crocodile holding grain in its mouth was firmly bound to the

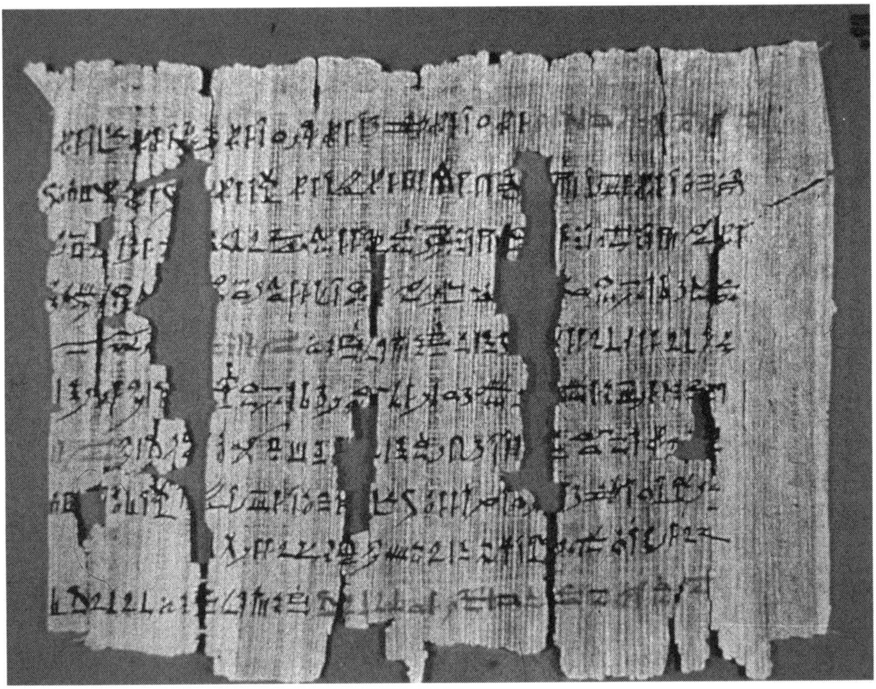

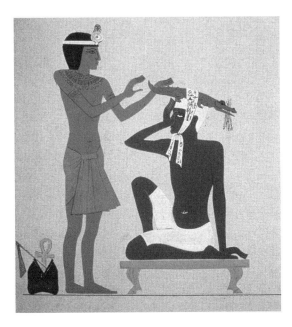

FIGURE 2-2A

The Ebers Papyrus.

FIGURE 2-2B

Headache treatment in ancient Egypt.

patient's head by a strip of linen inscribed with the names of the gods (Figure 2-2B). This may have produced headache relief by compressing and cooling the scalp.

Hippocrates described both the visual aura that can precede a migraine headache and its relief by vomiting in 400 B.C. He believed that headache could be triggered by exercise or sexual intercourse; that migraine resulted from vapors rising from the stomach to the head; and that vomiting could partially relieve the pain of headache. Plato believed that preoccupation with the body triggered headaches:

> *"Yes, indeed," he said, "this excessive care for the body that goes beyond simple gymnastics is about the greatest of all obstacles.... It is troublesome in household affairs and military service and ... it puts difficulties in the way of any kind of instruction, thinking, or private meditation—forever imagining headaches and dizziness and attributing their origins to philosophy.... It makes the man always fancy himself sick and never cease from anguishing about his body."*

Headache was believed to be inflicted by divine decree as a punishment for sins, and curable by repentance and good deeds. Celsius (215 to 300 A.D.) believed "drinking wine, or crudity [upset stomach], or cold, or heat of a fire or the sun" could trigger migraine. Aretaeus of Cappodocia (200 A.D.) is credited with first describing migraine headache.

The term *migraine*, derived from the Greek word *hemicrania*, meaning "half of the head," was introduced by Galen in approximately 200 A.D. He mistakenly believed it was caused by the ascent of vapors that were excessive, too hot, or too cold. Popular names that evolved over the years for this uncomfortable and often disabling disorder include *sick headache*, *blind headache*, and *bilious headache*.

A solution of opium and vinegar applied to the skin was widely used as a headache remedy in Europe during the thirteenth century. The vinegar probably allowed the opium to be absorbed more quickly through the skin. Vinegar compresses have also been used alone as a headache treatment. Shakespeare discusses headache treatment: Desdemona binds her husband's head with the handkerchief—a remedy still used by many migraine sufferers—that will later be her undoing:

OTHELLO: I have a pain upon my forehead here.

DESDEMONA: Faith, that is with watching; twill away again. Let me but bind it hard, within this hour. It will be well.

Erasmus Darwin, grandfather of Charles Darwin, suggested treating headache by centrifugation in the late 1700s. He believed headaches were caused by vasodilation and suggested placing the patient in a centrifuge to force the blood from the head to the feet. Fothergill introduced the term *fortification spectra* in 1778 to describe the typical visual aura or disturbance of migraine. Fothergill used the word *fortification* because the visual aura resembled a fortified town surrounded by bastions (Figure 2-3).

Liveing wrote the first book on migraine in 1873: *On Megrim, Sick-headache, and Some Allied Disorders: A Contribution to the Pathology of Nerve-storms*. This book originated the neural theory of migraine. He ascribed the problem to "... disturbances of the autonomic nervous system," which he called *nerve storms*.

William Gowers published an influential neurology textbook in 1888: *A Manual of Disease of the Nervous System*. Gowers emphasized the importance of a healthy lifestyle, a concept to which we have holistically returned, and he advocated treating headaches with a solution of nitroglycerin, 1 percent in alcohol combined with other agents. The remedy later became known as the *Gowers mixture*. Gowers was also famous for recommending Indian hemp (marijuana) for headache relief.

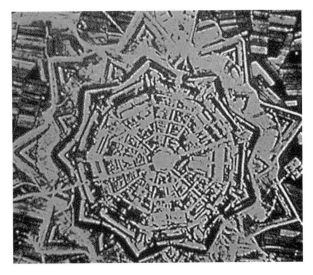

FIGURE 2-3

Fortification spectra: Aerial view of Palmonava, Italy.

Stephen King, the "horror" novelist, vividly describes the pain, sensory hyper-responsiveness, and feeling of prostration associated with migraine:

"…The headache would get worse until it was a smashing weight, sending red pain through his head and neck with every pulsebeat. Bright lights would make his eyes water helplessly and send darts of agony into the flesh just behind his eyes. Small noises magnified, ordinary noises as loud as jackhammers, loud noises insupportable. The headache would worsen until it felt as if his head were being crushed inside an inquisitor's lovecap. Then it would even off at that level for six hours. He would be next to helpless."

Firestarter, by Stephen King

Lewis Carroll described migrainous phenomena in *Alice in Wonderland* and *Through the Looking Glass,* depicting instances of *central scotoma* (blindness), tunnel vision, *phonophobia* (sensitivity to sound), vertigo, distortions in body image, dementia, and visual hallucinations (Figure 2-4).

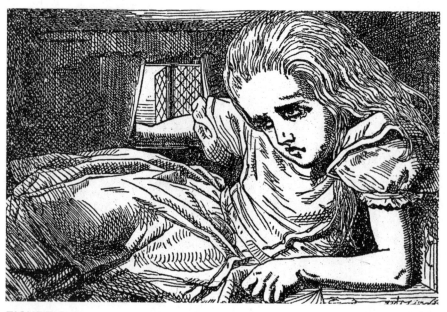

FIGURE 2-4

Alice in Wonderland.

Joan Didion describes a situation with which most headache sufferers can probably identify:

"We have reached a certain understanding my migraine and I. It never comes when I am in real trouble. Tell me that my house is burned down, my husband has left me, that there is gunfighting in the streets and panic in the banks, and I will not respond by getting a headache. It comes when I am fighting not an open but a guerilla war with my own life, during weeks of small household confusions, lost laundry, unhappy help, canceled appointments, on days when the telephone rings too much and I get no work done and the wind is coming up. On days like that my friend comes uninvited."

In Bed, by Joan Didion

Emotional well-being can produce a dramatic change in headache intensity. One dramatic example is found in the *Personal Memoirs* of Ulysses S. Grant. The general describes a sick headache he suffered on August 9, 1865. He attempts to cure it by "bathing [his] feet in hot water and mustard and putting mustard plasters on [his] wrists and the back of [his] neck." However, he gets complete relief only when he receives word that Robert E. Lee has agreed to discuss terms of surrender; "… the instant I saw the contents of the note I was cured."

In defining the elements of the *migraine personality,* Joan Didion's physician focuses on two areas that are usually considered to be areas of feminine concern—personal appearance and housework:

"You don't look like a migraine personality.… Your hair's messy. But I suppose you're a compulsive housekeeper.

Actually my house is kept even more negligently than my hair, but the doctor was right nonetheless; perfectionism can also take the form of spending most of a week writing and rewriting a paragraph."

In Bed, by Joan Didion

However, not all perfectionists have migraines, and not all migraineurs have perfectionistic personalities.

Migraine treatment advanced significantly in 1938 when John Graham and Harold Wolff demonstrated that the drug *ergotamine* worked by constricting blood vessels and used this as proof of the *vascu-*

lar theory of migraine. Ergotamine is produced from ergot, a fungus found on wheat and bread. Ancient Greek and Roman writings include references to "blighted grains" and "blackened bread," and to the use of concoctions of powdered barley flower to hasten childbirth. Written accounts of ergot poisoning first appeared during the Middle Ages (Figure 2-5). Epidemics were described in which the characteristic symptom was gangrene of the feet, legs, hands, and arms, often associated with burning sensations in the extremities—symptoms now recognized as ergot poisoning. The disease was known as *Ignis Sacer* or *Holy Fire* and, later, as *St. Anthony's Fire*, in honor of the saint at whose shrine relief was obtained. This relief may have resulted from the use of grain that was not contaminated during the pilgrimage to the shrine.

In 1853, Louis René Tulasne of Paris established that ergot was not a hypertrophied rye seed, but a fungus, *Claviceps purpurea*. Once infected by the fungus, the rye seed was transformed into a spur-shaped mass, purple-brown in color—the resting stage of the fungus known as the *sclerotium* (derived from the Greek *skleros*, meaning hard). The term *ergot* is

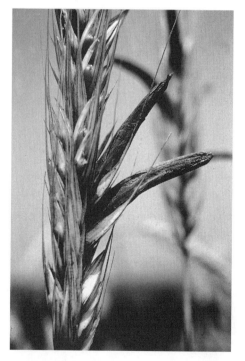

FIGURE 2-5

Ergot: fungus growth on rye.

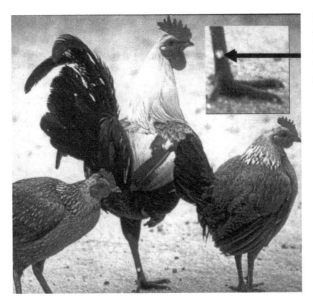

FIGURE 2-6

Ergot, the French word for rooster's spur.

derived from the French word *argot*, meaning *rooster's spur*, which describes the small, banana-shaped sclerotium of the fungus (Figure 2-6).

The use of ergot was romanticized by Alfred, Lord Tennyson (1809-97):

He gently prevails on his patients to try
The magic effects of the ergot rye.

The first pure ergot alkaloid, ergotamine, was isolated and used primarily in obstetrics and gynecology until 1925, when Rothlin successfully treated a case of severe and intractable migraine with a subcutaneous injection of *ergotamine tartrate*. This indication was pursued vigorously by various researchers over the following decades and was reinforced by the belief in a vascular origin for migraine and the concept that ergotamine tartrate acted as a vasoconstrictor. Dihydroergotamine (DHE®)* was synthesized by Stoll and Hofmann in 1943 and was used to treat migraine by Horton, Peters, and Blumenthal at the Mayo Clinic.

The modern approach to treating migraine began with the development of *sumatriptan* (Imitrex®) by Pat Humphrey and his colleagues.

---

*The brand names of medicines are in parentheses, throughout.

Based on the concept that *serotonin* can relieve headache, they designed a chemical that was similar to serotonin, although more stable and with fewer side effects. This development led to modern acute migraine treatment and to the elucidation of the mechanism of action of what are now called the *triptans*, seven of which are now available in the United States.

We are at the threshold of an explosion in the understanding, diagnosis, and treatment of migraine and other headaches. Many new treatments have been developed, and many more are in various stages of

> We are at the threshold of an explosion in the understanding, diagnosis, and treatment of migraine and other headaches.

development. Concomitant with this is the renewed dedication of clinicians to headache treatment and teaching. Let us hope that future headache sufferers will not relate to this refrain from *Iolanthe,* by W.S. Gilbert and Sir Arthur Sullivan (Love, unrequited, robs me of my rest [the nightmare song] 1882):

When you're lying awake with a dismal headache
And repose is taboo'd by anxiety,
I conceive you may use any language you choose
To indulge in without impropriety.

CHAPTER 3

The Causes
of Headache

CAUSES VERSUS TRIGGERS

IT IS IMPORTANT TO REALIZE the difference between a headache *cause* and a headache *trigger*. Among other things, stress and weather changes

> It is important to realize the difference between a headache *cause* and a headache *trigger*.

can trigger a headache. Knowing what *causes* a headache is crucial to treating the headache successfully. A brain tumor, a high fever, or head trauma can cause a headache (Figure 3-1).

Many people are convinced that their headaches are caused by certain foods. However, although many foods are recognized headache triggers, very few, if any, can directly cause a headache. One exception, of course, is the dreaded "ice-cream headache," in which ice cream or another cold stimulus to the back of the mouth produces a brief, severe headache.

TRIGGERS

Marie Alvarez suffered from two severe migraines a month for much of her life. They were severe and responded moderately well to treatment. In her 40s, she developed pain in the right front of her head that moved to the left and back of the head. She had a mild, chronic, nagging, left-sided headache, and then devel-

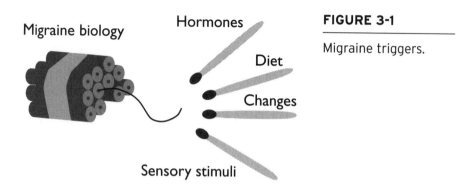

FIGURE 3-1

Migraine triggers.

oped neck pain. These migraines were much more frequent and difficult to treat. Eventually she was found to have a herniated disc in the upper part of her neck that was pushing on the nerve on the left side. She eventually had surgery, her headaches returned to their original location, and once again they became simple to treat.

This story illustrates an important concept. While all of Maria's headaches were migraine, a significant inciter or trigger made her new headache very hard to treat until it was located and corrected. A huge number of triggers exist (Table 3-1). Almost any kind of physical prob-

TABLE 3-1 Migraine Triggers

Diet

Hunger	Additives
Alcohol	Certain foods

Chronobiologic

Sleep (too much or too little)	Schedule change

Hormonal changes

Menstruation

Environmental factors

Light glare	Altitude
Odors	Weather change

Head or neck pain

Of another cause

Physical exertion

Exercise	Sex

Stress and anxiety

Letdown

Head trauma

lem in the neck or head, including the jaw joint (*temporomandibular joint disorder*), eyes, teeth, and neck, can be a trigger. Sometimes a worsening of migraine and, to a lesser extent, tension-type headache can be caused by physical illness, such as mononucleosis, thyroid disease, or sleep apnea; a chronic environmental factor, such as smells at work or chronic sleep deprivation; or a psychological condition, such as chronic stress or major depression. Unlike migraine, and perhaps tension-type headache, psychological conditions and other triggers play only a small role in making cluster headache worse.

On the other hand, triggers bring on headaches one at a time. For example, a person drinks a glass of red wine and a few hours later develops a migraine. The wine brought on a single headache, but it is not responsible for an overall worsening of the headache problem.

Types of Headache

Headache can be divided into two broad groups: *primary headache disorders* and *secondary headache disorders*. A *primary headache disorder* is one in which the headache itself is the problem. In other words, there is no deeper underlying cause. The most common primary headache disorder is *tension-type headache*; the second most common is *migraine headache*. The International Headache Society has classified the primary headache disorders, as shown in Table 3-2.

A *secondary headache* may be a symptom of an underlying condition, such as a brain tumor, stroke, or fasting. Secondary headache disorders can be ruled out by a thorough history and physical examination. Diagnostic testing may be necessary if suspicious features are present (see Table 4-1, Warning Signs—"Headache Alarms").

Most people who have headaches have a normal physical examination. Therefore, the history is the most important diagnostic tool the physician has at his disposal. Important diagnostic clues include when and under what circumstances the headaches began. For example, migraine and tension-type headaches usually begin in childhood or early adult life. The onset of a new headache after the age of 55 years is worrisome and could indicate a more serious disorder. Fever in associa-

TABLE 3-2   Primary Headaches

Classification
1. **Migraine**
   Migraine without aura
   Probable migraine without aura
   Migraine with aura
      Typical aura with migraine headache
      Typical aura with nonmigraine headache
      Typical aura without headache
      Familial hemiplegic migraine
      Sporadic hemiplegic migraine
      Basilar-type migraine
   Probable migraine with aura
   Childhood periodic syndromes that may be precursors to or associated with migraine
      Cyclical vomiting
      Abdominal migraine
      Benign paroxysmal vertigo of childhood
      Retinal migraine
      Complications of migraine
      Chronic migraine
      Status migrainosus
      Persistent aura without infarction
      Migrainous infarction
      Migraine-triggered seizures
   Migrainous disorder not fulfilling above criteria
2. **Tension-type headache**
   Infrequent episodic tension-type headache
      Infrequent episodic tension-type headache associated with pericranial tenderness
      Infrequent episodic tension-type headache not associated with pericranial tenderness
   Frequent episodic tension-type headache
      Frequent episodic tension-type headache associated with pericranial tenderness
      Frequent episodic tension-type headache not associated with pericranial tenderness
   Chronic tension-type headache
      Chronic tension-type headache associated with pericranial tenderness
      Chronic tension-type headache not associated with pericranial tenderness
   Probable tension-type headache
3. **Cluster headache and other trigeminal autonomic cephalalgias**
   Cluster headache
      Episodic cluster headache
      Chronic cluster headache
   Paroxysmal hemicrania
      Episodic paroxysmal hemicrania
      Chronic paroxysmal hemicrania
   Short-lasting unilateral neuralgiform headache attacks with conjunctival injection and tearing (SUNCT)

(continued on next page)

22

TABLE 3-2 Primary Headaches *(continued)*

Probable trigeminal autonomic cephalalgia
    Probable cluster headache
    Probable paroxysmal hemicrania
    Probable SUNCT
4. Other primary headaches
  Primary stabbing headache
  Primary cough headache
  Primary exertional headache
  Primary headache associated with sexual activity
    Preorgasmic headache
    Orgasmic headache
  Hypnic headache
  Primary thunderclap headache
  Hemicrania continua
  New daily persistent headache

tion with the onset of headache suggests an infection. Vigorous exercise or exertion, such as weight lifting, may trigger migraine. A person can have more than one type of headache, and the pattern may change over time. The most important headache is the one that causes the most pain or the greatest worry to the sufferer. Many doctors use questionnaires to help focus on symptoms and improve the reliability and efficiency of the history. In this way, the doctor will have more time for discussion, treatment, and teaching, and also to be sure that nothing of importance has been missed. While most headaches are not symptoms of a serious medical problem, some are. This is discussed in detail in Chapter 4.

LOCATION AND DURATION OF PAIN

A *unilateral* (one-sided) headache suggests migraine or cluster headache, or one of a few unusual types of headache. Migraine pain can change sides from one attack to the next or can involve both sides of the head. Cluster headaches are almost always one-sided, with the pain centered in or around the eye, temple, cheek, or adjacent areas. Tension-type headache typically involves both sides of the head. *Trigeminal neuralgia* is a disorder evidenced by jabs of brief, one-sided, severe pain (similar to an electric shock) on or near the upper or lower jaw or cheek that is triggered by light touch to a trigger zone. They may occur many times a day and last only a few seconds. Headaches caused by disease in the neck usually radiate from the neck to the back of the head on the side of the

> Establishing the headache profile is a critical factor in accurately diagnosing and appropriately treating headache.

disorder. In general, the location of pain in primary headache is not very revealing. Establishing the headache profile is a critical factor in accurately diagnosing and appropriately treating headache. Comments such as, "It hurts real bad for a long time" are not very helpful in finding the correct diagnosis.

FREQUENCY AND TIMING OF ATTACKS

Migraine attacks occur at various times—for example, in association with the menstrual cycle, on weekends, on vacation, when relaxing after stress, or at random. Cluster headaches usually occur in a regular pattern, typically one to three times a day during a cluster period, which usually lasts between two weeks and six months. The attacks occur at similar times of the day or night, often awakening the sufferer from sleep. Some brief-duration headaches occur dozens, and occasionally hundreds of times a day.

TABLE 3-3 How Long Does the Headache Last?

Headache Type	Typical Duration
Migraine	4 to 72 hours
Status migrainosus	Migraine lasting more than 72 hours
Cluster	15 to 120 minutes
Episodic tension-type	30 minutes to 7 days
Trigeminal neuralgia	Seconds

It is important for people with headaches to convey to their doctor how often their headaches occur. Sometimes they may only communicate the frequency and timing of their severe attacks, ignoring the more frequent or daily headache. This can lead to misdiagnosis and inappropriate treatment.

PAIN SEVERITY AND QUALITY

The severity of the pain and the speed of its onset and resolution are also important diagnostic clues. Headaches of sudden onset are worrisome. Doctors often use a 1 to 10 scale, with 1 representing minimal discomfort and 10 the most excruciating pain the person has ever experienced. Migraine pain and cluster pain are often rated as 10/10. The absolute number used is not particularly important, although people who often say that their headache is "15/10" tend to damage their credibility. What is most helpful is consistency, so that both the patient and the physician can tell if progress is being made in treatment.

Migraine pain is characteristically pulsating or throbbing, but it can begin as a dull, steady ache that slowly evolves. It may not acquire a throbbing quality until the pain becomes more severe. Cluster headache pain is deep, boring, or piercing—described as feeling as though a red-hot poker were being thrust into the eye. Generally, tension-type headaches are dull, band-like, or vise-like.

Associated Features

Nausea, vomiting, and even diarrhea can occur during a migraine attack. *Photophobia*, an unusual or heightened sensitivity to light, and *phonophobia*, a heightened sensitivity to sound, can also be associated with migraine. Eye-tearing, redness, congestion of the nose on the side of the headache, and swelling of the face are seen predominantly in cluster headache.

Aggravating and Relieving Factors

As noted above, headaches often have triggers, and many people confuse triggers with causes. For example, you might get pain after pulling a muscle in your shoulder or neck and then get a migraine-like headache. The neck pain would be the trigger of the migraine. There may be other migraine triggers, but when the neck problem is serious, the migraine will be much more severe. Removing the trigger is important, but it is also important not to get confused and say that the problem is strictly in the neck. Persons with trigeminal neuralgia have trigger points on the face and the mucous membranes of the mouth. Slight stimulation of these trigger points by eating, speaking, exposure to cold air, brushing the teeth, or stroking, shaving, or washing the face may provoke an attack. Menstruation is a regular trigger of migraine in many women. Wine can be a migraine trigger—strangely white wine triggers migraine in France and red wine is a trigger in England. In Italy, everything seems to trigger a headache.

Sleep problems may be a cause or a trigger of headaches. Sleep apnea, a condition in which an individual stops breathing while asleep and then partially awakens, is a common problem, especially in the overweight individual. It may cause morning headache. Some psychological disorders, such as depression, may make it difficult to fall asleep or stay asleep.

Life-style stresses abound. These include marital and family status, education, occupation, outside interests, friendships, and major life changes, such as marriage, divorce, separation, a new job, retirement, or a birth or death in the family. Employment provides many stressors. Is the person's work satisfying or merely drudgery? Is there conflict in the workplace? Exposure to drugs or toxins in the workplace may trigger headaches. Workers in munitions factories may develop nitroglycerin headaches, and carbon monoxide exposure due to poor ventilation can trigger headache.

Behavior during the Headache

Many people find that sleep will clear their attacks and migraineurs often retire to a dark, quiet room and lie motionless to obtain relief. Relief can sometimes be obtained by applying hot or cold compresses or pressing on the arteries of the scalp, but only during the period of compression. Migraine frequency and severity often decrease during the last two trimesters of pregnancy or with the onset of menopause. Tension-type headache sufferers may seek to distract themselves and remain active, or they may seek relaxation or rest. People with cluster headache find that sitting upright, rocking in a chair, pacing to and fro, or engaging in vigorous movement lessens the pain.

FAMILY HISTORY

Some headache disorders run in families. Approximately 50 to 60 percent of migraineurs have a parent with the disorder, and as many as 80 percent have at least one first-degree relative with migraine disorder. Cluster headaches rarely occur within the same family. Nearly half of those with tension-type headaches have family members with similar headaches.

Familial headaches do not necessarily imply a genetic factor, although this often seems to be the case with migraines. Shared environmental exposures may also cause familial headaches. For example, a malfunctioning furnace may cause carbon monoxide-induced headaches in an entire family.

Past Headache History

Past response to a particular treatment may support a particular headache diagnosis, although a specific headache treatment can mask a serious neurologic disease. Treatment failure may be the result of the wrong dose or not allowing enough time for a potential benefit to accrue, such as stopping or discontinuing a preventive headache medication after only a one-week trial. The successes and failures of past treatment may improve future treatments, helping the doctor to better select subsequent therapies. Medication-induced or rebound headaches can result from the excessive use of nonprescription pain relievers, such as aspirin or acetaminophen, as well as narcotics, barbiturates, ergots, and triptans.

Individual Impact of Headache

Diagnosis alone does not provide enough information. Headaches differ in severity and affect an individual's ability to function. The Migraine Disability Assessment (MIDAS) questionnaire assesses the impact of headache on work and school, chores, and household work, as well as

> Headaches differ in severity and affect an individual's ability to function.

social, family, and leisure activities. It measures actual days of missed activity—for example, work absenteeism and the number of days with high levels of activity limitation. It can help both doctors and patients focus on how headaches affect a person's life. Migraine is the likely diagnosis when there is a high level of disability due to a primary headache that is recurrent (comes and goes). A MIDAS score greater than 10 indicates significant disability. Another impact test is called the *Headache Impact Test (HIT)-6*. It is a little different in that it assesses emotional impact as well as physical disability.

PHYSICAL AND NEUROLOGIC EXAMINATIONS

After obtaining a thorough history, a physical examination is performed. It should include the taking of vital signs, including pulse, blood pressure, and a baseline weight, examination of the heart and lungs, and listening to the blood vessels in the neck, such as the carotid and, perhaps, vertebral arteries, for turbulent blood flow. The head and neck should be examined for growths, bruises, thickened blood vessels, trigger points, or other tender areas. The jaw should be examined for tenderness, decreased movement, asymmetry, or severe "clicking." Neck rigidity may be due to irritation of the lining of the brain and might suggest *meningitis*, masses in the skull, or hemorrhages.

When performing the neurologic examination, the doctor may look for swelling of the nerves in the back of the eyes (*papilledema*), which suggests increased pressure around the brain that warrants a test to rule out a mass lesion, such as a brain tumor. Arm or leg weakness, or facial paralysis (known as *focal neurologic deficits*) may indicate brain disease. A thickened or nodular scalp artery, diminished or absent artery pulsations, reddened, tender scalp nodules, or necrotic lesions of the scalp or tongue suggest *giant cell arteritis* (also called *temporal arteritis*), a cause of headache and sudden blindness in the elderly.

Sometimes a diagnosis cannot be made on the first visit, and sometimes the initial diagnosis is incorrect. A headache diary can be extremely helpful in uncovering unrecognized patterns and providing clues to diagnosis. The diary can be used to log headache frequency, severity, and duration, the medications that were used, and possible headache triggers.

Diagnostic Testing

Most people with headaches do not need tests to establish their diagnosis. Diagnostic testing is done to identify serious underlying diseases, such as stroke, brain tumor, or *subdural hematoma*. Diagnostic testing can also establish a baseline for drug treatment, reveal reasons to avoid certain drug treatments, such as an unexpected illness, and measure drug levels to determine how much of a drug has been absorbed into the body.

Some features of the headache or characteristics of the sufferer may suggest a need for diagnostic testing and may indicate the need for emergency treatment (see Chapter 4).

Some factors suggest that headaches are not due to an underlying organic cause. When the factors listed in Table 3-4 are present, there is less of a need to investigate a headache.

TABLE 3-4   Reassuring Headache Factors

- Regular or near-regular hormonal timing of the headache
- Appearance of headache after sustained exertion
- Relief with sleep
- Food, odor, or weather changes provoking headache

Specific Tests

Laboratory tests are not necessary for diagnosis in a typical, healthy migraineur or someone who is experiencing tension-type or cluster headache, but they may be helpful prior to treatment. They are used to rule out more serious disorders, of which headache is occasionally a symptom. An *electrocardiogram* (EKG) may be needed when there are risk factors for heart disease, or to establish a baseline prior to the use of triptans, ergots, or other vasoconstricting drugs. Physicians often request liver function tests prior to using drugs that may affect the liver, and a complete blood count (CBC) and chemistry profile before starting some types of preventive treatment. A sedimentation rate measures inflammation in the body and can establish the diagnosis of giant cell arteritis. Unexpected or overused medications that have a direct effect on headache and its treatment can be identified by means of drug screening and toxicology studies. Routine testing for Lyme disease is not recommended. However, serum antibody testing may be needed if an individual who has never had a headache develops one, or a headache is accompanied by other manifestations of Lyme disease.

Electroencephalography

This test measures the electrical activity of the brain and is an excellent test for epilepsy. The American Academy of Neurology has determined that an electroencephalogram (EEG) is not useful in the routine evaluation of people with headache. Migraine aura symptoms and epilepsy symptoms are sometimes similar, in which case an EEG may be used to establish the correct diagnosis.

Computed Tomography and Magnetic Resonance Imaging

Computed tomography (CT) uses a computer to analyze multiple X-rays in order to produce better images. In contrast, magnetic resonance imaging (MRI) uses a computer, a powerful magnet, and radio waves to analyze the area of the body in question. CT and MRI are not needed in people with migraine if there has been no recent change in the headache pattern, no history of seizures, and no focal neurologic findings. CT and MRI are useful when headaches are atypical and do not fit into any defined primary group of headaches—for example, they are used to rule out the possibility of a brain tumor (see Chapter 4).

Magnetic Resonance Angiography and Magnetic Resonance Venography
Magnetic resonance angiography uses the MRI machine to examine arteries. It is a screening tool for suspected aneurysms (weakened areas of blood vessel that pouch outward) or *arteriovenous malformations* (abnormal tangles of vessels). Magnetic resonance venography looks for evidence of a blood clot or obscuration in the veins or sinuses that drain blood from the brain. These *sinuses* are very different from the sinuses of the nose (Figure 3-2).

Lumbar Puncture
A lumbar puncture (see Figure 3-3), also called a *spinal tap*, involves placing a needle between two vertebrae in the lower back and into a pocket that contains the cerebrospinal fluid. This test measures the pressure of the fluid and determines whether or not infection or inflammation is present. The lumbar puncture is crucial to diagnosis in the five clinical situations listed in Table 3-5.

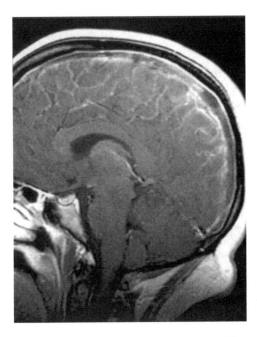

FIGURE 3-2

Magnetic resonance venography: An MRI of the brain showing cerebral veins and venous sinuses.

TABLE 3-5   Situations in which Diagnostic Lumbar Puncture Is Indicated

- The first or worst headache in a person's life
- A severe, rapid-onset, recurrent headache
- A progressive headache (over days or weeks)
- An atypical, chronic intractable headache
- A daily headache with symptoms of high spinal fluid pressure
- A new type of headache accompanied by a fever

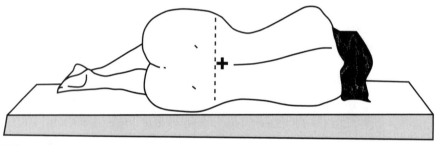

FIGURE 3-3

Patient in position for a lumbar puncture.

A lumbar puncture may need to be done even if the CT or MRI is normal, because these tests may miss the presence of blood or infection, and they cannot diagnose increased spinal fluid pressure. People with daily headaches of recent onset, particularly those whose immune system is weakened, may have chronic meningitis, the meningitis of Lyme disease, or meningitis of cancer cells, all of which require lumbar puncture for diagnosis.

THE CONCEPT OF PRIMARY HEADACHE

Primary headache disorder is a condition in which the headache is not caused by another disease or medical condition, but is a disorder unto

The most common primary headache disorder is tension-type headache; the second most common is migraine headache.

TABLE 3-6   Summary Regarding Diagnostic Tests

1. Diagnostic tests can help to exclude organic headache caused by structural abnormality of the brain, head, or neck, or by another illness that causes headache. They can also identify other important conditions that should be considered during treatment.
2. Electroencephalography is not helpful in the evaluation of recurrent headache.
3. Lumbar puncture is crucial in diagnosing people who are experiencing their first or worst headache and those with severe, sudden-onset headache, progressively worsening headache, atypical chronic intractable headache, or headache accompanied by fever and stiff neck.
4. Computed tomography or magnetic resonance imaging is not routinely needed in adults with migraine or episodic tension-type headache. Neuroimaging should be considered if headache alarms are present, the headache pattern has significantly changed, the neurologic examination is abnormal, or seizures occur.
5. Specific testing, such as magnetic resonance imaging, computed tomography, or lumbar puncture, is appropriate prior to beginning treatment if the person is at risk, the treatment poses a risk, or worrisome clinical features are present.
6. Consultation and additional testing are often indicated for people with thunderclap headache, chronic daily headache, headache associated with focal neurologic signs, fever, severe neck stiffness, or headaches beginning after age 50.

itself. The most common primary headache disorder is tension-type headache; the second most common is migraine headache. Secondary headaches are caused by another problem or condition. Of the secondary headache disorders, fasting headache (a headache precipitated by hunger) is the most common, followed by headache due to nose/sinus disease or head trauma.

The concept of primary headache is an interesting one. It appears that the brain can spontaneously produce pain and then take it away. Some experts have even called primary headache a "reflex." Migraine and other primary headaches can be thought of as part of a larger group of benign, recurrent conditions, including premenstrual syndrome (PMS), cyclic vomiting in childhood, and some cases of recurrent vertigo in adults.

Why would nature cause so many people to have recurrent pain unrelated to injury? Experts have speculated that some primary headaches may be normal pain reflexes gone awry—a human form of the fright response to threat that causes animals to become inactive—or a warning that the environment is too stressful. Nature does not do what is comfortable for the individual, but what is good for the species.

Perhaps there is an advantage to some individuals being highly sensitive to serve as an early warning system that something is amiss in the environment. In some people, this "reflex" has simply gotten out of hand and become dysfunctional for both the individual and society. These are only speculations at this time, but they may ultimately prove fundamental to understanding the nature of primary headache.

THE CONCEPT OF SECONDARY HEADACHES

Secondary headaches are due to an acquired injury, an infection, or a malformation of the brain present since birth. Once the cause is identified, it is treated, and if the treatment is effective, the headache goes

> Secondary headaches are due to an acquired injury, an infection, or a malformation of the brain present since birth.

away completely. This idea is simple and very much the way we like to view illness: you treat an infection and the symptoms go away, permanently; you cure the tumor and there is no more headache.

In some cases, a secondary headache is very much like a primary headache. A person with viral meningitis may have a throbbing headache with nausea and vomiting and may, in fact, temporarily respond to a *migraine-specific* medicine.

Finally, some people have been cured after a secondary headache disorder, such as meningitis, but continue to have a chronic headache problem that is very similar in its symptoms to primary headache problems, including chronic tension-type headache and chronic migraine.

WHEN YOU VISIT YOUR PHYSICIAN

If you are seeing your doctor about your headache—especially if you are seeing a specialist—bring the following to your appointment:

1. A headache calendar that covers at least one month, if possible
2. The most recent CT or MRI of your brain or neck, or a copy of the reports if the test(s) was normal
3. Copies of your most recent blood tests
4. Your last EKG, if you have had one in the last five years
5. A list of your prior acute and preventive headache treatments
6. A list of all your current drugs and food supplements
7. Any prior consultation reports

CHAPTER 4

Serious Headaches Requiring Medical Attention

"**O**H MY GOD! THE PAIN! My head feels like it's going to explode! I hope it's not a brain tumor!"

Fears of brain tumor, aneurysm, or other unknown, but equally dire consequences usually cross the mind of someone who experiences a first severe headache. With all the media attention these dramatic diseases garner, it would be unusual if these thoughts did not intrude. Fortunately, such incidences are rare. Primary headaches (headaches that are themselves the problem) greatly outnumber secondary headaches (headaches that indicate an underlying problem). Headache is rarely the first indication of a dangerous medical condition. But what if it is? When should you definitely seek immediate help? Table 4-1 lists a series of warning signs that will help you identify serious problems.

SERIOUS MEDICAL CONDITIONS THAT CAN CAUSE HEADACHE

Aneurysm

One of the most serious illnesses of which headache is a symptom is called a *subarachnoid hemorrhage*—bleeding under the membrane that surrounds the brain. A subarachnoid hemorrhage is usually caused by a weakening of the walls of a blood vessel, causing a bulge called an *aneurysm*. If the aneurysm breaks, blood rushes onto the surface of the brain. Sometimes the blood vessel that breaks is part of an abnormal tangle of blood vessels called a *vascular malformation*. The headache caused when a blood vessel

TABLE 4-1 Warning Signs—"Headache Alarms"

- Sudden-onset or "thunderclap" headache
- A marked change in headache pattern, such as increased frequency, intensity, or duration
- Neurologic signs and symptoms, such as double vision, blindness, confusion, dizziness, weakness, or sensory loss
- Signs of irritated brain surface, such as a severely stiff neck (a sign of meningitis), or sudden spike of pain with quick movement of the head
- Symptoms of brain damage, such as weakness on one side of the body
- Symptoms of a new generalized illness, such as an unexplained fever
- History of a known serious disease that can involve the head or brain, such as acquired immune deficiency syndrome (AIDS) or cancer
- Persistent or unexplained vomiting
- Nontrivial head trauma or convulsions
- Relentlessly worsening headache over days or weeks
- Blood pressure higher than 180/115
- You are 50 (or older) and you just started having headaches

Other Reasons to See Your Doctor

- You feel so bad you cannot go to work or enjoy yourself
- Your headaches last for days
- Nonprescription drugs rarely provide relief
- You get headaches with exercise

breaks comes on very suddenly, similar to being hit with a baseball bat. Sometimes, but rarely, aneurysms come on more slowly, but they will still reach peak intensity in about 60 seconds. Aneurysm bleeds are true medical emergencies. A significant percentage of people die before reaching the hospital. Many will die or suffer a stroke even with the best care. Early diagnosis and, in some cases, early surgery can save lives and prevent future strokes. Unless the aneurysm is surgically clipped or a coil placed within it through the artery—and even if the person appears healthy after an aneurysm has bled—it may bleed again, perhaps fatally (Figure 4-1).

Giant Cell Arteritis

Giant cell (temporal) arteritis is a disease that usually occurs in the elderly. It causes inflammation of blood vessels in the head. This condition

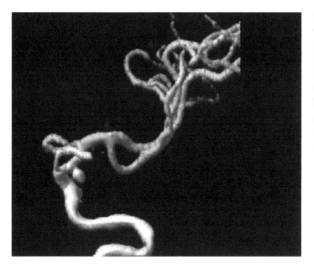

FIGURE 4-1

An aneurism is a bulge in the wall of a blood vessel (lower left). This kind of image is used by neurologists to rule out other diagnoses than migraine.

may be associated with scalp tenderness over an artery, a generalized feeling of illness, and joint and muscle pain (which is part of a condition called *polymyalgia rheumatica*, which is very common in people with giant cell arteritis), low-grade fevers, depression, and visual disturbances or stroke.

Meningitis and Encephalitis

Meningitis is an infection of the spinal fluid and the linings covering the brain. There are several types of meningitis, the most dangerous of which is *bacterial* meningitis. The person is usually very ill and has an extremely stiff neck, a severe headache, a fever, and sometimes reduced consciousness and seizures. Treatment with antibiotics should be begun as quickly as possible because long-term complications may be avoided with early treatment. Individuals who have *viral* meningitis are usually less ill and have fewer complications. The headache in meningitis is two-sided, generally severe, and worsens relentlessly over hours or days. The neck is often so stiff that the person has trouble bending the neck forward more than a few inches. The headache may be accompanied by sensitivity to light and sound, as well as nausea and vomiting. A mild jolt, such as hitting a small bump in the road when riding in a car, is extremely painful.

Encephalitis is an infection involving the substance of the brain, not just the coverings. Symptoms such as reduced consciousness, weakness, and speech and language problems are more prominent than in meningitis. The most famous encephalitis of late is caused by West Nile virus, but there are many different infectious causes. Meningitis and, at times, encephalitis require a spinal tap for diagnosis, as well as a computed axial tomographic (CT) scan or magnetic resonance imaging (MRI).

Brain Tumor

Headache caused by a brain tumor can resemble any type of primary headache, but it especially resembles migraine or tension-type headache. A brain tumor can also cause worsening of a primary headache problem. It used to be believed that a headache that occurs upon awakening is typical of a brain tumor, but the fact is that this is uncommon, and morning headaches are usually *not* caused by brain tumors. Headache is not the most reliable sign of brain tumor. More important symptoms of brain tumor include weakness, loss of vision or sensation on one side of the body, clumsiness of the limbs, difficulty walking, and seizures that are due to dysfunction of the part of the brain where the tumor is located (Figure 4-2).

Sometimes people with brain tumors have a headache that starts out mild, but relentlessly worsens over days or weeks. This type of headache may also be caused by blood clots that press on the brain. More than half of those with brain tumors have headache, and 80 percent of them have pain on the same side as the tumor. However, brain tumor headache is usually associated with weakness, trouble talking or walking, or seizures. People with brain tumors may have headaches (which are often mild) that resemble migraine or tension-type headache. These headaches often become progressively worse, start late in life, or are associated with seizures, confusion, prolonged nausea, hemiparesis (one-sided weakness), swelling of the nerves in the back of the eyes, or other neurologic abnormalities.

Pseudotumor (a condition that looks like a tumor but *is not*) occurs when there is elevated spinal fluid pressure, usually accompanied by

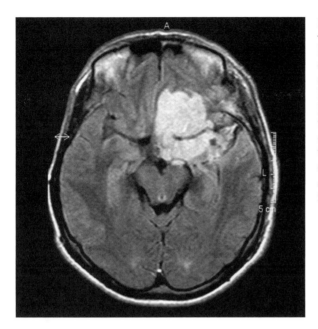

FIGURE 4-2

MRI is used in the diagnosis of a number of disorders of the brain. The MRI on the left shows a brain tumor (circular light-colored area), which in this case was the cause of headache and other neurologic symptoms.

signs of swelling in back of the eye and temporary visual symptoms. This type of headache is relieved by a spinal tap—some people even ask for another one!

Hypertension

A common misconception is that headaches are caused by high blood pressure. In order for high blood pressure to cause a headache, it has to be so high that it overcomes the normal protective reflex of the brain's blood vessels. While the point at which this occurs varies, usually the diastolic blood pressure (bottom number) needs to be above 115. Blood pressure so high that it causes a headache is a medical emergency. Some people may have high, but not immediately dangerous, blood pressure due to pain caused by a headache. Some blood pressure medicines can treat migraine, and a headache may occur when a person's blood pressure medicine is stopped, if the particular medication was helpful for the headache. Likewise, treating high blood pressure with medicine that also treats migraine may help the headache, giving the impression that high blood pressure causes headache.

Dissection

A *dissection* is a rupture of the lining of an artery. Blood enters and expands the wall of the artery, narrowing or completely obstructing the artery and limiting blood flow to the brain. A headache resulting from dissection may resemble migraine, even migraine with aura. It may cause transient stroke-like spells or a full-blown stroke—a sudden loss of neurologic function that persists for more than 24 hours. Symptoms include weakness, numbness, blindness, and the inability to speak (Figure 4-3).

Complicating this picture is the fact that migraineurs are at increased risk for developing a dissection. Minor neck injuries, including falls, car accidents, chiropractic manipulation, and even roller coaster rides, can precipitate dissection.

SPINAL HEADACHE AND OTHER LOW PRESSURE HEADACHES

As discussed in Chapter 3, a spinal tap (lumbar puncture) is a procedure in which a doctor collects spinal fluid through a needle placed into the spine in the lower back. It is a very safe, minor surgical procedure, with

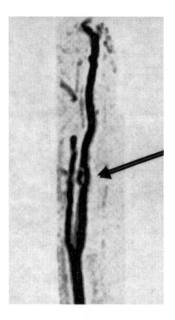

FIGURE 4-3

A carotid dissection is a rupture of the lining of the carotid artery, which limits the supply of blood to the brain and can cause a headache that resembles migraine.

long-term complications and permanent injury being extremely rare. However, about 10 percent of the time, a medium-term complication called a *spinal headache* occurs. This headache may be caused by a persistent leak of spinal fluid through a hole in the coverings of the spinal cord. The headache goes away when the sufferer lies down, but will return in seconds or minutes when he stands up again. It usually starts in the back of the head or upper neck and spreads over the entire head. Nausea and light and sound sensitivity do not accompany this type of headache. Lying down flat for hours after a lumbar puncture, which is commonly recommended, does not protect someone from getting a spinal tap headache.

Spinal headaches usually improve over several days. During this time, the sufferer should lie flat and drink plenty of fluids. An abdominal binder may help. Rapidly administered oral caffeine (No-Doz®) may help; intravenous caffeine is more effective. A procedure called a *blood patch*, in which the person's own blood is withdrawn from the forearm and injected into a space surrounding the spinal cord, may need to be done. This procedure is 98 percent successful and works instantly.

CHAPTER 5

Managing Headaches:
An Overview

A PHYSICIAN MUST TAKE CHARGE and be very firm about treatment when someone has a burst appendix, but the patient assumes a passive role until it is time for rehabilitation. Headache treatment should be a

> Headache treatment should be a two-way street, with the patient communicating a goal and desires about his headache management, the doctor contributing her knowledge and values, and the final plan incorporating both perspectives.

two-way street, with the patient communicating a goal and desires about his headache management, the doctor contributing her knowledge and values, and the final plan incorporating both perspectives.

Probably the single most important thing that you and your doctor can do to ensure success in treating your headaches is to maintain open channels of communication. Education about headache and its treatment is as important as any medication. When you receive a diagnosis, you should thoroughly understand what is meant, the implications of that diagnosis, what your symptoms mean, and what you can do to improve your situation. Your treatment plan should consider your diagnosis, your symptoms, and your lifestyle.

This, however, does not put full responsibility on the healthcare professional to compensate for your lifestyle. He may recommend lifestyle changes to decrease or eliminate your headaches. This may be as small a change as walking, getting a neck massage, or practicing breathing and relaxation techniques at the first twinge of a headache. All of these have been effective for some people. You may be advised to follow a consistent program of walking, cycling, swimming, or aerobics classes to reduce the severity and frequency of your headaches. You have to be willing to implement the recommended changes.

A headache sufferer may arrive at the doctor's office expecting an immediate diagnosis and rapid treatment and cure. A common complaint heard in headache centers from first-time patients is, "I spent all day there; I had a bunch of tests; I filled out a dozen forms; and I don't feel any better." Unfortunately, headache control takes time and sometimes a good deal of trial and error. Tests will not make you feel better, but they may help the doctor understand how to improve your condition.

Part of the responsibility of a conscientious physician is to help you to better understand your headaches by demystifying the problem and laying the groundwork for the job ahead. It is also to teach you what you need to know to be able to manage the problem safely and effectively at home.

The physician may not—in fact, should not—explain it all at once. It is almost impossible to retain information when too much is discussed in a single office visit. Table 5-1 outlines the information that should be conveyed to you at the first or second visit.

If your problem is a primary headache disorder, you need to know that at some point, testing will stop and treatment will begin. People with primary headaches often search endlessly for a *cause* of their headaches and end up dissatisfied. Once the necessary workup is completed, it is best to accept the fact that the headache is a primary one.

TABLE 5-1 Critical Information for Headache Sufferers

- The difference between a primary and secondary headache, and what type of headache you have
- The difference between a benign and an ominous headache
- The difference between a trigger and a cause of headache
- The biological basis of the headache

Blame and anger can greatly worsen your headache. You and your doctor need to roll up your sleeves and get to work, because while treatment may be simple and effective, it could require many treatment trials before a satisfactory solution is found.

A necessary first step may be to stop taking too much pain medication. A person who has daily headaches often becomes very upset when the doctor makes this suggestion. The patient might believe that the doctor thinks he is addicted, but there is a very big difference between *rebound headache*—headache caused by overuse of acute headache medication—and addiction. Addicts are trying to escape from society or emotional pain. In general, people who are rebounding want to take care of their families, do their jobs, and be part of society. Thus they begin the vicious cycle of taking more and more medicine to continue functioning. Rebounders have to understand that even if their motivations are excellent, rebound is an unhealthy behavior. No matter how noble the reasons, rebound must stop.

Work with your doctor to establish realistic goals. If you want your headache to be gone in five minutes and feel dissatisfied with anything that works more slowly, you will probably never be satisfied. For example, once a headache has become moderate or severe, the best oral treatments have a 3 in 5 chance of relief at two hours and a 1 in 7 chance of relief at 30 minutes. That means that 6 of 7 people do not have relief at 30 minutes, and a much smaller proportion of them are actually pain-free. Outcomes improve greatly if the headache is treated in the mild stage, but it can by no means be in the "pain-free-in-five-minutes level" for most people. Also, no medicine will work every single time. For some people, treatment will be successful 95 percent of the time, for others 80 percent of the time, and a few unlucky people might find that the best they can do is find a treatment that works half of the time.

Try to establish realistic expectations about side effects for both acute and preventive medicines. Most headache medicines have side effects. You may have to tolerate side effects and work with them. Your doctor can choose medicines that may have fewer side effects or medicines with less bothersome side effects—for example, if you suffer from insomnia, you might choose a medicine that causes nighttime sleepiness.

If you suffer from primary headache, you should realize that your headaches may be controlled, but you will not be cured. In studies of preventive medication, only half of the participants get 50 percent or more relief of their headaches with the first drug taken. In an office setting, doctors can often do better than this by individualizing treatment. With preventive treatment, headache improvement is not immediate: it usually begins in about four weeks, and it generally takes about eight weeks before you can be sure the preventive treatment is working. You may be told that you might have to tolerate some side effects and not to throw away any new medicine for at least two weeks. To minimize dissatisfaction, doctors and patients can use helpful strategies, such as once-a-day (as opposed to more frequent) dosing and taking medication at night, if sleepiness or other side effects are caused by the treatment.

You should communicate your preferences. For example, your worst headaches might only be treatable at the cost of sleepiness. Maybe you would prefer to bear the pain and stay awake; maybe you would prefer to have less pain and be a bit sleepy. Some people will take the pain and not the medicine; others will take the side effects to obtain relief.

The doctor/patient relationship is a partnership. Family members can be helpful, but they are not critical members of the treatment partnership. The doctor should, as much as possible, deal principally with

> The doctor/patient relationship is a partnership.

the patient, not the spouse, mother-in-law, or concerned friend. Interested family members may be invited—by you—into the doctor's office and allowed to ask a few questions, but it is usually not appropriate for them to give most of the history or answer most of the questions. (Obviously this does not apply when the patient is a young child or is mentally or psychologically incapacitated.)

Take charge of your care as much as possible. Know your medicines, including how often you take them. Know the parts of your treatment plan that do not include the use of medications and how you should implement those other aspects of the plan. This helps to simplify treatment and puts you in charge of your own health and life.

To fully participate in a partnership with your doctor, be prepared to answer the basic questions she needs to know in order to manage your treatment. Your doctor needs to know the frequency, duration, and intensity of your headaches, and might ask questions such as:

- When did you first start having headaches?
- What is the timing of your headaches—time of day, or before or during your menstrual cycle?
- Do your headaches come and go, and does the pain move from one spot to another?
- How long does a headache usually last?
- Do you have a headache virtually every day?
- Where do you feel pain—one side of your head, both sides, behind one eye, or the front of your head?
- Does the pain creep up and get worse, or does it slam you suddenly?
- How does the pain feel—dull ache, throbbing, mild, or excruciating?
- What other symptoms do you have with your headaches?
- Do you feel nauseated or vomit?
- What medications or other solutions have you tried, and did these provide any relief?
- Do you take any vitamins or herbal supplements?
- Do you get a headache when you skip meals or eat certain foods?
- Do your headaches follow physical activity, such as sex or exercise?
- Have you noticed a connection between extreme stress and the start of a headache?
- Have you noticed anything that seems to make the pain worse when you have a headache?
- Have you had any kind of head trauma, such as a car accident or sports injury?
- Do others in your family have headaches?

Whether or not you choose to keep a headache calendar, you should anticipate these questions and be prepared to answer them to the best of your ability. Also, you must be very honest about the extent of your headache disability and medication use. It is absolutely vital that there is no confusion about this between you and your doctor. Your doctor may use a tool, such as the MIDAS (discussed in Chapter 1), to fully understand your headache issues (see Figure 5-1).

Add up numbers 1 through 5. If the total is 5 or less, you have minimal or infrequent disability often with low treatment needs, but if you have infrequent, severe, disabling headache, you may benefit from aggressive treatment. If the total is 6 to 10, you have mild or infrequent disability and moderate treatment needs. If the total score is 11 to 20,

---

FIGURE 5-1 Migraine Disability Assessment*

PATIENT'S NAME:_____

DATE OF BIRTH:_____ /_____ /_____   DATE:_____ /_____ /_____

INSTRUCTIONS: Please answer the following questions about ALL of the headaches you have had over the last 3 months (90 days). Write your answer in the box next to each question. Write zero (0) if you did not do the activity in the last 3 months.

1. How many days in the last 3 months did you miss work or school because of your headaches?	DAYS ☐ ☐
2. How many days in the last 3 months was your productivity at work or school reduced by half or more because of headaches? (Do not include days you counted in question #1 where you missed work or school.)	DAYS ☐ ☐
3. How many days in the last 3 months did you *not* do household work because of your headaches?	DAYS ☐ ☐
4. How many days in the last 3 months was your productivity in household work reduced by half or more because of your headaches? (Do not include days you counted in question #3 where you did not do household work.)	DAYS ☐ ☐
5. On how many days in the last 3 months did you miss family, social, or leisure activities because of your headaches?	DAYS ☐ ☐
6. On how many days in the last 3 months did you have a headache? (If a headache lasted more than one [1] day, count each day.)	DAYS ☐ ☐
7. On a scale of 0 to 10, on average how painful were these headaches? (Where 0 = no pain at all and 10 = severe pain.)	_____

MIDAS categories 0-5

*Modified from the MIDAS Questionnaire

you have moderate disability and urgent treatment needs, and if the total is 21, you have severe disability and urgent treatment needs. Those with MIDAS scores higher than 5 should see a physician. If your job is at risk due to headaches, some very aggressive treatments may be reasonable. This type of informational chart encourages these important discussions between you and your doctor.

It is necessary to understand the difference between an *acute* and a *preventive* medicine when discussing the effects of medication. You should know your acute medication limits in order to prevent rebound, and realize that if you are treating a headache with medicine every day, the headache problem is likely to eventually become much worse.

People look at their own health in terms of three types of *locus of control*, the things that determine health. One is the extent to which the doctor is in control, the second is the extent to which we control our own health, and the third is the extent to which random, chaotic factors affect our health. Realistically, all three factors are important. People who view their health as principally determined by the doctor or by chance do not do as well as those who have a more balanced locus of control.

Headache sufferers need structure and balance. For many of them, a structured world without extremes or variability is the ideal. You can control stress—thereby moving your locus of control toward "self"—but do not expect to eliminate it completely. Exercise in moderation and make sure that each day includes pleasurable activities and moderate food and alcohol intake. In general, strive to have a balanced lifestyle. Practice daily some form of stress-reducing technique, such as meditation, journalizing, breathwork, or yoga. These measures may guide you toward a less stressful lifestyle, or at least help you move in that general direction. You have to take the lead in modifying your lifestyle. Your physician can help you identify the aspects of your lifestyle that may be contributing to your headaches, but you must make a realistic compromise between the ideal and the other demands on your life.

Trigger identification requires good doctor/patient communication. There is considerable evidence that stress, sleep, hormones, and, to some extent, weather can trigger headache. There is evidence that some, but not many, food triggers are actually important in headache development. Sometimes people develop false, but very firmly held beliefs about the role that food triggers play in their headaches. These are often people who have headaches nearly every day, which makes identifying food or other triggers nearly impossible. Very rarely, they will need to go on an elimination diet in which they eat almost nothing but boiled rice for a number of days. If this does not control the headaches, it is reasonable to assume that food triggers are not a significant factor.

Keeping a headache calendar is a useful tool for both diagnosis and treatment. The calendar is used to record the duration and severity of your headaches, and their response to treatment. You should record on your calendar not only the medication you take for your headaches, including the dosage and what time you took it, but nondrug therapies as well. Be sure to record any changes or innovations you make in exercise, mealtimes, and your sleep habits in an attempt to improve your condition. Your doctor needs to know these things to treat you effectively, so be honest! Do not record when you meant to exercise, or when you meant to go to bed. Record what you actually did, and when you did it!

It is an excellent idea to keep your calendar for a few months before seeing a headache specialist for the first time. After a while, maintaining a calendar may no longer be worthwhile, as most of the information it can yield has already been identified. Some people will give their headache calendar such extreme attention that the headache takes on a more prominent role than necessary.

Smoking cessation and exercise are beneficial. Aerobic exercise is most effective, and exercise that causes an increased pulse rate should be done 3 to 4 days a week for at least 20 minutes. Mechanical disturbances of the neck and jaw may worsen headache, and mechanical changes that eliminate or lessen stress on the neck (moving the computer screen or changing your chair at work) or jaw (not chewing gum) may be helpful. For those whose headaches worsen with aerobic exercise, walking can be very beneficial.

Exercise is good for your general health. It can reduce anxiety and muscle tension and make you feel refreshed. It may make you more flexible (especially if you stretch), condition your heart, and increase your energy level and ability to focus. Regular exercise, good health practices, regular mealtimes, adequate sleep, and maintaining accustomed patterns of activity are all of benefit to headache sufferers, for whom it is more difficult to adjust to changes in expected external stimuli, such as mealtimes, stress, and awakening and retiring times.

Movement increases your brain's production of *endorphins*, natural hormones that fight pain, and exercising three times a week for 30 to 45 minutes can help reduce headache frequency. Figure out which forms of exercise work for you and discontinue or modify the ones that trigger headache. Remember to keep well-hydrated.

As far as possible, it is best to adhere to a regular routine, seven days a week. Get up and go to bed at approximately the same time every day. Eat your meals at about the same time every day, and eat about the same amount of food, especially at breakfast, when it is easy to vary widely on weekends. Sunday brunch can be tempting, but a break in routine can result in a headache.

Avoiding or managing headache triggers can also be effective, especially in combination with other therapies.

THE MIND/BODY CONNECTION

There is an unproven, but *fundamental* doctrine that any severe psychological problem, such as depression or anxiety, will make headache diffi-

There is an unproven, but *fundamental* doctrine that any severe psychological problem, such as depression or anxiety, will make headache difficult to treat.

cult to treat. Stress is the most common trigger for headache, and biofeedback and relaxation can be very helpful. Some people need medicines and/or psychological management of depression or anxiety, or they simply will not get better. It does not matter if the headache itself causes the depression or anxiety—once it has started, it has to be treated.

FAMILY RELATIONS

Family relations can be an important part of a headache problem and headache management and treatment. There should be a balance of support. Family and friends can be either overinvolved in the headache patient's disorder or underinvolved to the point of being neglectful. Sometimes families will assume "it's just a headache," such as one (usu-

> Family relations can be an important part of a headache problem and headache management and treatment.

ally much less severe) that they have had themselves. In other families, overinvolvement with the headache problem does not allow the headache sufferer to be distracted from his problem. This dynamic can also interfere with the person's ability to take charge of his own care. The family may undermine the treatment by demanding further tests and studies, even though such studies are time-consuming, expensive, and counterproductive to the treatment plan. Support groups can be valuable because the headache sufferer can choose his own level of involvement (see appendix).

TREATMENT OVERVIEW

It is useful to divide headache treatments into those that include the use of medication and those that do not (see Table 5-2). If you rarely have headaches, you may not need the treatments indicated in every box below, but if you have a severe, significant headache problem, your doctor will probably ask you to try something listed in each treatment box. When you visit your doctor, you may discuss each of the four areas of treatment, decide whether they need modification or improvement, and

TABLE 5-2 Examples of a Headache Treatment Plan

MEDICINE	NO MEDICINE
Acute	**Body**
Nonsteroidal anti-inflammatory drugs for moderate headache.	Vigorous walking 3 times per week.
Triptan for more severe headache.	
Preventive	**Mind**
Increase dose of amitriptyline from 50 to 75 mg at night.	Biofeedback with relaxation training.

reassess each area of treatment at the next visit. These treatments are discussed in detail in subsequent chapters.

Is Your Doctor Skeptical about Your Headaches?

Signals that you need to find another doctor include:

- She looks confused or uninterested while you are describing your headache symptoms
- He says you have to learn to "deal" with the headache
- Your physician does not answer your questions
- Your physician rushes you and immediately suggests a pain medication
- An existing medical problem leads you to believe that you would benefit from seeing a headache specialist
- You take nonprescription medications almost every day, and your doctor does not suggest a plan for you to come off these medicines
- Your doctor tells you that she does not feel comfortable trying to diagnose and treat your severe headaches. (On the other hand, a second opinion is okay.)

HOW TO FIND A GOOD HEADACHE DOCTOR

Ask your friends and family (especially those who also have headaches). Call a friend who is a physician, nurse, or other health care professional in your area.

Call a local medical center or university and ask for the doctor-referral service. Then, pose this key question: "Could you give me the names of three doctors who are headache specialists in this area?"

An excellent referral source is the American Council for Headache Education (ACHE), the American Headache Society's patient education organization. Its website (www.achenet.org) lists the physicians in your state who are members of the American Headache Society.

When looking for a headache specialist, ask if the doctor:

• Is board-certified or board-eligible.
• Is well-credentialed, including belonging to professional headache organizations, such as the American Headache Society.
• Frequently treats people who have headaches.
• Takes courses and participates in continuing medical education that keeps him abreast of new developments in diagnosis and treatment.
• Publishes papers on headache and teaches others about headache.

COMBATING STUMBLING BLOCKS
SET UP BY INSURANCE COMPANIES

Insurance companies often seem more interested in denying appropriate care than in supplying it. They may try to restrict access to specialists, inpatient hospital care, and medicines that may be necessary for you to get control of your headaches. To combat this:

• You can ask for a referral to a headache specialist. If your primary care physician gives you a medication for your symptoms and it does not work, and you go through the same routine with him a second or third time, you probably need to see a specialist.
• You can ask your doctor to send a "letter of medical necessity." If your health insurance company limits the number of migraine pills it will pay for in a given month, your doctor may need to send a letter of medical necessity to the insurance company explaining what has been tried, over what time period, what worked and what did not, and why you need more medication.

Many insurance companies deny biofeedback and stress management, or have made their reimbursement so low that there are no caregivers in their plans who have the training or inclination to teach these types of headache management skills. This is a difficult problem, and you might have to "bite the bullet" and pay for these services out-of-pocket. Ask your mental health practitioner if he provides this type of therapy in a group setting at a reduced rate.

Primary Headache— Migraine

CHAPTER 6

Migraine: The Big One

"I've had headaches all my life," the woman sitting in the waiting room said, "but they're not migraines. I don't know if this doctor can do anything for me or not."

"How do you know they're not migraines?" her companion asked.

"Well, with migraines, I read that you get a kind of warning. You know, flashing lights in front of your eyes and things like that."

"I sure do! I can always tell when I'm going to get a headache."

"Not me! It just hits me out of the blue. And do I get sick! My mother was the same way, and my grandmother, too. I'm afraid this is going to be a big waste of time."

WHEN IS A HEADACHE A *MIGRAINE*? There is no known cause for migraine and no test for it. For years, even headache experts argued about what makes a migraine a migraine. Finally, in the 1960s,

> There is no known cause for migraine and no test for it.

a group of experts, "the Ad Hoc Committee on Classification of Headache," came up with a one-paragraph description of what constitutes a migraine headache:

"Recurrent attacks of headache, widely varied in intensity, frequency, and duration. The attacks are commonly unilateral in onset; are usually associated with loss of appetite and, sometimes, with nausea and vomiting; in some (patients they) are preceded by or associated with conspicuous sensory, motor, and mood disturbances; and they are often familial."

For about 20 years, this was the accepted definition of a migraine. Headaches that were usually one-sided, that sometimes seemed to cause stomach upset, and that were *sometimes* preceded by warning signals, such as flashes of light, dizziness, or changes in mood, were called *migraines*. By the early 1980s, doctors from the International Headache Society (IHS) decided they needed a better way to diagnose migraine. They separated migraine into several types, the most important of which were migraine without aura and migraine with aura. These had previously been called *common* migraine and *classic* migraine.

Migraine Without Aura

The first speaker in the conversation at the beginning of this chapter probably suffered from common migraine, or migraine without aura (see Table 6-1). The IHS defines migraine without aura as headaches that last for a defined period of time, usually hours. They have no known secondary cause, and neurologic examination is generally normal. The headache itself must have a number of symptoms from the list in Table 6-1, but it does not need to have all of them. In addition to pain, the headache sufferer needs to have nausea with or without vomiting, or sensitivity to light and sound to be diagnosed as having migraine.

Migraine was referred to as *sick headache* for years, and many people still use this phrase. This is most likely due to the nausea that occurs in

> Migraine was referred to as *sick headache* for years, and many people still use this phrase. This is most likely due to the nausea that occurs in over 70 percent of migraineurs.

TABLE 6-1 Migraine Without Aura

Previously called *common migraine*

Description: The headache, when untreated—or treated, but without improvement—lasts from 4 to 72 hours, and at least two of the following characteristics are present:

1. The headache is on only one side.
2. There is a pulsating quality.
3. The pain is moderate or severe and interferes with normal daily activities.
4. The pain is aggravated by walking stairs or similar physical activity.

During the headache, at least one of the following is present:

1. Nausea and/or vomiting.
2. Photophobia (light sensitivity) and phonophobia (sound sensitivity).

The headache is not caused by any other disorder.

---

over 70 percent of people with migraine—also called *migraineurs*. Usually the pain is aggravated by movement. Although migraine is thought of as one-sided, almost 40 percent of the time the pain occurs on both sides of the head. It often starts as a mild, nonthrobbing headache that starts to throb as the pain becomes more severe. Many people are sensitive to light and sound during a migraine, and some are sensitive to odors. (Figure 6-1).

Many people with migraine report sinus congestion. In fact, most people with "sinus headache" actually have migraine and do not have an identified disorder in the nasal passages or sinuses. Similarly, many migraineurs report upper neck pain that can occur before, during, or after the headache pain.

Mary first developed severe, one-sided headaches with nausea at around age 14, and they occurred a half dozen times a year throughout high school. They had increased to twice a month by the time she finished college. She now is at her first job and is getting severe headaches three times a month. She also gets what she calls regular *headaches. Aspirin works for the regular headaches, but almost never helps the severe ones. She misses work due to headaches once a month.*

Mary suffers from migraine without aura. The headaches started a few years after her first period, and they will probably be with her in various forms until after menopause. Since seeing a headache specialist, she has

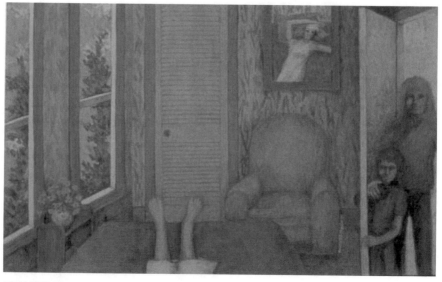

FIGURE 6-1

Serving Time by Nancy Ellen Wheeler, time away from the family.

learned to take her prescribed *abortive* medication as soon as she feels a headache coming on and she is usually able to "head off" the migraine. She also takes a *preventive* medicine every day, whether she has a headache or not. Her doctor prescribed 400 mg of vitamin B2 daily, and she noticed a decrease in the number of headaches. She could not take such a high dose of vitamin B2 when she was pregnant, and her headaches increased.

MIGRAINE WITH AURA

Migraine with aura is the official name for a headache preceded by a physical warning, which can be as mundane as tiny "floaters" in front of

Migraine with aura is the official name for a headache preceded by a physical warning, which can be as mundane as tiny "floaters" in front of your eyes or as dramatic as hallucinations.

your eyes or as dramatic as hallucinations. They normally last about 20 minutes.

Ronald experienced a 20-minute visual problem on four occasions in the last year. He suddenly noticed a small spot that grew larger, then disappeared. The spot was surrounded by shimmering blue lights. He experienced this three times on the right side and once on the left. A mild headache occurred after the visual disturbance, but it lasted only half an hour. His neurologic examination was normal.

Ronald suffers from migraine with aura. Although he has unusual features—the headache is trivial, color is unusual, and the light portion of the aura is not very prominent—this could be little else but migraine aura. After his doctor discovered he had a family history of migraine, Ronald was sent home with reassurance. A brain scan was not necessary. He knows to pull over when he has an aura while he is driving.

Another type of migraine with aura is *basilar migraine*. In this type of headache, the aura that usually precedes the headache includes double vision, spinning dizziness (also known as vertigo), ringing in the ears, extreme unsteadiness in walking, or changes in level of consciousness, even fainting. While this kind of migraine may occur at any age, it tends to be more common in teenage girls.

Tammy, a 17-year-old girl, was in physics class when she had what her friends described as a spell. Staring at the blackboard, she began seeing double. This lasted for about a minute. She began to feel like the room was spinning and then she passed out. Although her panicked friends insisted that she was unconscious for at least 10 minutes, her teacher told the EMTs it was not more than three by his watch. When she awoke, she said her head hurt "terribly, all over," and she began to vomit. She was very unsteady on her feet when she tried to walk. This passed in a few minutes, but the headache lasted for hours. She was taken to the emergency room, where she was observed for several hours and discharged. Two weeks later, she had a second attack.

Tammy suffers from basilar-type migraine, also called *Bickerstaff Syndrome*. This syndrome is benign and although it may occur a few more times, and is admittedly frightening, it is unlikely to be a severe problem. She may develop other types of migraine in later years.

THE CAUSE OF MIGRAINE

Migraine has long been recognized as a serious problem. For years, doctors and scientists have tried to discover the cause and offer relief. From

> From the nerve storms of the 1870s to the vascular theory popular in the 1950s, many causes of migraine have been postulated.

the nerve storms of the 1870s to the vascular theory popular in the 1950s, many causes of migraine have been postulated. Unfortunately, some of these persist today, preventing a more complete understanding of headaches among both doctors and the public.

You may hear a lot about *serotonin* and migraine. This theory was developed in the 1970s. It was believed that migraine was due to an imbalance in serotonin function. Serotonin is a neurotransmitter, one of many small molecules used to transmit impulses from one nerve to another. There was certainly evidence to this effect. However, none of these were enough to serve as a test for migraine.

In the 1990s, the neurogenic inflammation theory suggested that migraine was due to inflammation of blood vessels and the lining of the brain. Currently, the neurovascular theory is the best theory. It suggests that migraine is an underlying brain disorder that affects the blood vessels. The nerve endings are responsible for much of the pain of migraine. However, migraine involves much more than head pain, and most of the other symptoms are brain-derived (Figure 6-2).

We have learned a great deal about what migraine is, but we do not have a final answer. When we do find the answer, it will probably be that migraine is not caused by any single factor. There will be different types of migraine, different genetic backgrounds, different ways in which the symptoms develop, and perhaps even a variety of sources for the pain, all resulting in a final manifestation with somewhat similar symptoms shared by individual sufferers.

Normal **During a Migraine**

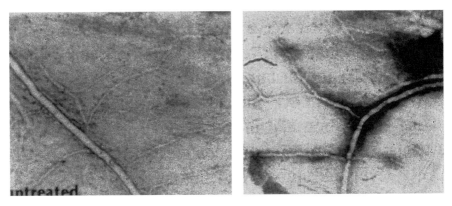

FIGURE 6-2

Blood vessels leak fluid during a migraine attack as a result of chemicals being released from nerve endings.

Five Things We *Do* Know about the Cause of Migraine

We definitely know five things about the cause of migraine, but there is no agreement on a single way that migraine is produced. It may be that migraine is not one problem and that, in fact, it has multiple causes.

Fact one: The brains of migraineurs are hyperexcitable and behave differently than the brains of nonmigraineurs. Migraineurs see a flash of light when exposed to a magnetic pulse, but it was recently discovered that migraineurs see this flash at a significantly lower power pulse than do nonmigraineurs. This shows that the visual part of the migraineur's brain is hypersensitive. Another difference is the brain's response to recurrent stimuli. Migraineurs have more excitable visual and sound systems. If migraineurs are shown an alternating checkerboard over a period of time, the amplitude of their brain wave response tends to increase, whereas nonmigraineurs tend to show a decrease in the amplitude of this wave as they get used to it (Figure 6-3). Similar changes in normal brainwave pattern are observed when migraineurs listen to a series of clicks.

Fact two: The aura of migraine is caused by a wave of increased electrical activity that moves across the surface of the brain, followed by loss of activity (Figure 6-4). Accompanying the excitation is a brief peri-

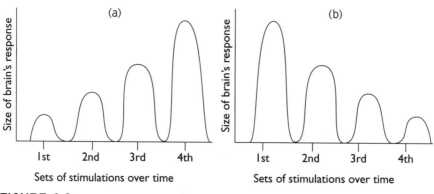

FIGURE 6-3

People with migraine are more sensitive to visual stimuli. (a) The migraine sufferer's response to a series of visual flashes increases in intensity over time, whereas (b) a normal person's response to the same series of flashes decreases over time.

od of increased blood flow, then a period of decreased blood flow that is not caused by contraction of a blood vessel. The band of increased brain activity causes the bright lights seen in typical visual aura. The migraineur experiences a corresponding movement of the bright part of

> The aura of migraine is caused by a wave of increased electrical activity that moves across the surface of the brain, followed by loss of activity.

visual hallucination as the activated area travels across the brain. In the wake of this activated area of the brain, there is diminished brain function. This causes visual loss—either a gray, dark, or white area that the person cannot see through.

Fact three: One or more areas of the brain that are specific for migraine are activated during a headache. The first such area has been called the *migraine generator*, although it has not been proved whether it is a generator of migraine. This area of the brain is in the upper brainstem (see Figure 6-5) and is likely to be very important because it receives input from emotional and sensory areas and sends impulses

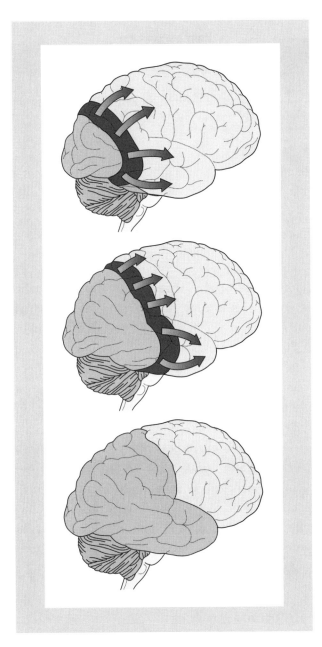

FIGURE 6-4

The migraine aura is associated with a wave (black) of increased electrical activity and blood flow followed by decreased electrical activity and blood flow.

back to these areas. Fibers carrying pain information reach the centers of the brain in this area, and the areas of the brain thought to be the migraine generator have connections with the pain centers that receive information from the blood vessels.

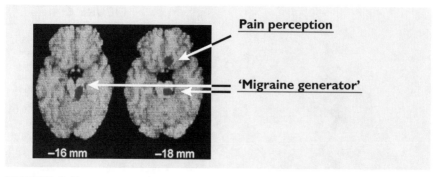

Pain perception

'Migraine generator'

−16 mm   −18 mm

FIGURE 6-5

This study shows blood flow changes in the brain stem during a headache. Blood flow increases in the areas indicated with arrows, possibly causing the headache.

Fact four: An inflammation of the covering of the brain (the *meninges*) or blood vessels causes the throbbing pain of migraine. Mechanically or electrically stimulating the blood vessels and meninges results in inflammation. The nerve endings of people who have migraine have been shown to secrete inflammatory proteins around meninges and vessels. The blood vessels dilate and leak, and the nerve endings on the blood vessels and meninges become more reactive. This results in the throbbing pain that many people associate with migraine.

Fact five: People who have migraine attacks often develop sensitivity to normally nonpainful stimulation of the scalp or other parts of the head and sometimes even the arm; this is called *allodynia*. Most commonly, the sufferer experiences it as scalp sensitivity and also has increased pain with bending, straining, or shaking the head. Allodynia develops after the migraine starts, usually one to four hours later. Once allodynia is established, migraine is much harder to treat (see Table 6-2).

How Common Is Migraine?

Migraine is a common disorder. Migraine occurs in approximately 12 percent of the U.S. population. The first American Migraine Study, published in *JAMA* in 1992, showed that 17.6 percent of women and 6 percent of men had experienced one migraine attack in the previous year.

TABLE 6-2 Symptoms of Allodynia

• Tenderness of scalp
• Tenderness of muscles on head or neck
• Pain when brushing hair
• Hates cold wind in hair
• Heat from stove bothers headache
• Takes off jewelry; loosens collar

Migraine occurs in approximately 12 percent of the U.S. population.

The second American Migraine Study, done 10 years later, had similar (in fact, slightly increased) numbers (18.2 percent in women and 6.5 percent in men) (Figure 6-6).

Migraine throughout Life

Migraine tends to start earlier in boys (around age 10) than in girls (around age 15). In children, it is more common in boys than girls, but after puberty, it is much more common in girls.

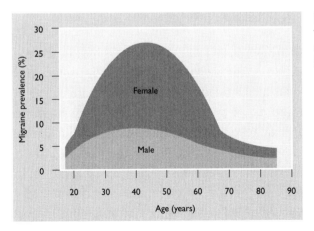

FIGURE 6-6

Age and sex distribution of migraine.

In women, it is most common between ages 40 and 45. Men tend to have migraine at a slightly younger age. This means that it tends to strike people in their economically most productive years, and this is a big part of the effect that migraine has on society. In the United States, in any given year, 13 percent of people have migraine and many fail to treat it. Migraine is the cause for many days of missed work, and it undeniably has a negative effect on the careers of many individuals.

Migraine can occur at any age. Even very young children are suspected of suffering from migraine, although diagnosing them is almost impossible until they learn to speak. Parents may report that their child

> Migraine can occur at any age.

has attacks during which he becomes pale, stands in his crib, cries, vomits, and then goes to sleep and wakes up comfortable and cheerful. A year or two later, when the child is able to talk, he will indicate that his head is painful during these attacks.

Severe nausea with migraine tends to diminish in the elderly, and aura is more likely to occur without a headache, prompting the name "migraine equivalents of the elderly." These attacks can imitate a *transient ischemic attack* (TIA), a warning spell for a stroke. Sometimes tests and even hospitalizations result when a migraine is mistaken for a TIA.

SYMPTOMS OF MIGRAINE

In order to understand all the symptoms of migraine, it is best to use the broadest conception possible—*complete migraine*, which includes four stages: the prodrome, the aura, the headache, and the postdrome.

The premonitory symptoms, or *prodrome*, can occur from hours to one day before the actual headache. The prodrome may involve a large variety of nonpainful behaviors and feelings. People may be sluggish or depressed. They may experience food cravings and increased appetite. In fact, food cravings directed by a person's preferences may explain why chocolate is often falsely identified as a trigger of migraine. Mood

In order to understand all the symptoms of migraine, it is best to use the broadest conception possible–*complete migraine*, which includes four stages: the prodrome, the aura, the headache, and the postdrome.

changes, often irritability, are common prodromes. Yawning is yet another prodrome.

Migraine aura is reported by about 20 percent of migraineurs. It occasionally occurs with every headache, but more often it accompanies only some headaches. There are many kinds of auras. The most common aura is the visual aura, and the most typical visual aura is the *scintillating scotoma*. This aura generally starts just off center, to the right or the left of the individual's area of central vision. A bright area of flashing lights expands over about 20 minutes to cover a significant portion of the visual field on one side (Figure 6-7). The bright lights are most typically short, flashing lines in a herringbone pattern. The lights are usually white or yellow, but they may be a variety of other colors. As the scintillation migrates across the visual field, it may leave in its wake a *scotoma*, an area of decreased vision that is seen as black, gray, white, or clear. Visual migraine auras are often not perfectly typical, as described

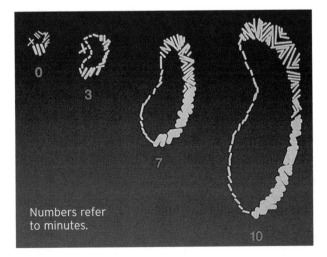

Numbers refer to minutes.

FIGURE 6-7

Scintillation scotoma is the most common aura seen with migraine, and enlarges with time.

above. They may be bilateral, travel from the outside to the inside, or even switch sides during a single attack. Often patients report that the visual problem is only in one eye. While it is possible that a visual problem originates in the eye (*retinal* migraine), this type of aura is thought to be very rare. To best investigate a visual aura, alternately cover each eye and fixate on a point in the middle of a blank piece of paper or on the wall. Observe what parts of your visual field are affected and then draw what you see for each eye. Repeat this process every few minutes to map out the changes in the aura over time.

The second most common type of aura is the sensory aura, during which a feeling of tingling or numbness occurs for about 20 minutes (Figure 6-8). The numbness typically begins in one hand or near the lips on one side. It generally spreads or grows in the area of the body involved, or it may jump from the face to the hand or vice versa.

Other auras may involve a loss of the ability to speak normally (*aphasia*), weakness on one side of the body, or the hallucination of abnormal smell. One rare type of aura that is more common in children

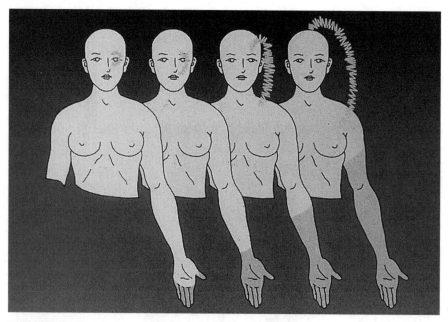

FIGURE 6-8

Visual and sensory auras grow during a migraine.

than adults involves visual distortions and alterations in perspective and body image. It has been called the "Alice-in-Wonderland Syndrome," based on the imagery in Lewis Carroll's novels. In fact, Lewis Carroll may have gotten his ideas for his books from his own auras.

Bobbi, a 41-year-old woman with a long history of migraine, recalls peculiar spells during childhood. From the age of 4 to 17, she would get spells that were entirely related to her hearing: "Every sound around me—speech (my own and that of others)—would assume the same overpowering rhythm." There was nothing she could do about it. She remembers being terrified of the spells when she was very young, but she eventually became accustomed to them and would lie down until they went away.

Her most striking spells were of the Alice-in-Wonderland variety. "On many occasions, particularly while reading, I would suddenly feel that my body had grown from the waist up, and that I was looking down at my book from a distance of 10 feet or more. I distinctly remember this happening semi-regularly when I was about 20. It has happened since, but it is a relatively rare thing. At about the same time, I was riding my bike one day and lost half my field of vision. This never occurred again." The spells were not associated with headache, but she developed severe migraine headaches without auras after age 20.

❊ ❊ ❊

Holly, a 23-year-old woman, has unusual seizure-like spells associated with her migraines. They can occur as often as twice a day and last 20 minutes to 2 hours, but "time is meaningless; it could be a second or days." The right side of her face becomes numb ("You could stick a pin into it"), and her tongue feels very thick, as if it were filling her mouth, making it difficult for her to speak. Her eyes flutter and her balance is off. The day before or the morning of an attack she will typically say, "It's not going to be a good time today." She had at least one episode of confusion: while driving in the neighborhood where she grew up, she suddenly became disoriented; she had no idea of where she was or how long she had been there.

She had an unusual spell when she was a college student. She woke up feeling tired and feverish. She took her temperature, and it went from 99° to 104° within an hour. Four days later, she had a headache that she described as feeling as if she had been struck by a lightning bolt or a volcano had erupted inside her head and she was unable to speak. A friend found her lying on her bed with her legs upright against the wall, and said, "You're climbing the walls!" She was able to spell out numbers on her hands but not talk.

The most striking episode occurred while she was in college. A "little space man" took her into a "little spaceship." She could see her body lying like a dead weight on the bed beneath her while her mind and all that was essentially her *floated in the air above her body. A friend walked into the room, could not rouse her, and summoned the campus emergency team. The static of their walkie-talkies pulled the spaceship back to earth, and when the ship attempted to rise, it was pulled back by the static. She was not frightened; she felt that she was in a "better place." When she awoke, everything was blurry; the movements and expressions of the people around her seemed both slower and exaggerated. She described a friend's smile as "ripping right across her face."*

Both these women suffer from very unusual migraine aura. No one would make a diagnosis and accept it without testing. However, with repeated negative testing, over time, the women themselves became certain these spells all were migraine symptoms.

Auras can occur one after another. A person might first experience a typical visual aura, followed by a sensory aura, then an aphasic aura,

> Auras can occur one after another. A person might first experience a typical visual aura, followed by a sensory aura, then an aphasic aura, and finally, a motor aura.

and finally, a motor aura. Some people have a time gap between the end of the aura and the beginning of the headache. During this time interval, thinking processes are generally not normal, although it is difficult to characterize them specifically.

The next phase of migraine is the headache itself. Usually it is very similar to migraine without aura: throbbing, pulsating, or severe pain on one side that gets worse with movement, along with nausea, vomiting, and increased sensitivity to light and sound. Often, however, the pain is on both sides of the head and does not always throb. Other symptoms may occur. These include pale, clammy skin and an absence of normal stomach activity. Some headache patients vomit undigested stomach contents hours after their headache begins. Migraineurs may retain fluid during a headache, and their fingers, feet, and faces may be slightly swollen. A vari-

> A variety of thinking and behavioral problems may accompany migraine.

ety of thinking and behavioral problems may accompany migraine. These include difficulties with concentration and memory, slight declines in alertness, and a tendency to use the wrong word or change letter order when writing. Migraineurs usually exhibit "hibernation behavior" during severe headaches; they want nothing more than to crawl away into a cave.

During a headache, a person may experience brief flashes of light called *phosphenes,* that last seconds and may shoot or streak across the visual field. As previously discussed, another symptom experienced during a headache is allodynia, sensitivity to otherwise pleasant or non-painful touch. Many migraine patients state that their "hair hurts" and that they cannot brush their hair during a severe attack. Others have trouble laying the painful side of their head on a pillow, prefer not to wear jewelry or tight collars, avoid air blowing on the head, or avoid heat or cold applied onto the scalp. This sensitivity usually starts near the site of maximal pain, but then travels to the other side of the head or even down the neck to the arm.

Some migraine sufferers note that their headaches end in a specific way. There may be an elimination of a large amount of urine, a bowel movement, or perhaps an increase in vomiting, followed by an abrupt sense of release in the head with an easing of pain over a few minutes. Occasionally, a sufferer will say, "I wish I could vomit and get over my headache." Some patients even induce vomiting to relieve severe headache.

After the headache comes the *postdrome,* which often involves feelings or sensations that are out of proportion to the severity of the pain.

> Progress is being made, and someday the "magic bullet" for migraine may be found.

These often include feelings of depression and tiredness. There may be unusual joy, or even a manic state that is more than would be expected from simple relief that the headache is gone.

The Future of Migraine Treatment

Research into the causes and treatment of migraine is ongoing. Progress is being made, and someday the "magic bullet" for migraine may be found. In the meantime, staying abreast of the most current theories and treatments will ensure that you are receiving the best possible treatment for your headaches. Joining organizations, such as the American Council for Headache Education (ACHE) (phone: 856-423-0258; website: www.achenet.org) and local support groups, can be an important part of educating yourself about your particular affliction.

Basilar Migraine

As illustrated earlier in this chapter in the example of Tammy, a 17-year-old girl with migraine with aura, spells of basilar migraine can present a confusing picture. The symptoms can be quite dramatic, and can mimic other far more serious illnesses. The word itself is misleading: *basilar* implies a *vascular* mechanism, but these events are now believed to be *neural*, rather than vascular.

In basilar-type migraine, the aura may be two-sided and can lead to temporary blindness. This visual aura is usually followed by *ataxia* (severe incoordination), *vertigo*, ringing in the ears, double vision, nau-

> In basilar-type migraine, the aura may be two-sided and can lead to temporary blindness.

sea and vomiting, jerky eye movements, slurred speech, pins and needles on both sides of the body, or a change in level of consciousness and thinking. The aura often lasts less than one hour, is usually followed by a headache, and, although the symptoms can be upsetting, is nothing more than migraine with an aura clinically localized to the brainstem.

Basilar migraine was once considered mainly a disorder of adolescent girls, but it affects all age groups and both sexes, just as migraine does.

Migraine Equivalents

At different ages, children may suffer repeated attacks that last hours or even days. They may develop repeated spells of neck twisting (*torticollis*) at about age two. Children a little older may get abdominal migraine with attacks of abdominal pain and vomiting that resolve completely. Adults may get attacks of spinning dizziness (vertigo) that last hours or days and disappear spontaneously, or respond to preventive migraine medication. Older adults get auras without any headache or with only minimal head pressure. When an aura is not followed by a headache (particularly in mid or late life), it is considered a migraine equivalent.

Menstrual and Hormonal Aspects of Migraine

Migraine often begins—or increases dramatically—when a woman enters puberty and generally improves after menopause. This is due to

> Migraine often begins–or increases dramatically–when a woman enters puberty and generally improves after menopause.

the fact that the sex hormones *estrogen* and *progesterone* have an effect on migraine. Many women tend to get their most severe or only migraines around the time of their period. The most distinctive form of menstrual migraine occurs just after the onset of flow and appears to be due to the sudden drop in estrogen that occurs around the menses. The brain's abnormal response to normal hormonal fluctuations determines whether a woman will develop menstrual migraine. Replacing estrogen reduces the occurrence of these migraines.

Some women have premenstrual migraine headaches associated with premenstrual syndrome. Many women who suffer regularly from migraine report that the migraines around or during their periods are the worst ones. Other than the timing, the only things that differentiate menstrual migraine from ordinary migraine are the severity and the poor response to treatment that some women have. Not all menstrual migraines are resistant to treatment, however. Many women have menstrual headaches that are no more difficult to treat than any other headaches.

Although, in general, migraines get better several years following menopause, some women report that their headaches worsen during menopause. Hormone replacement therapy using estrogen may also help this kind of headache. Many other factors need to be taken into account in any decision to replace estrogens after a natural menopause.

Migraine Patterns Related to Time

The time of day, month, or year may have an effect on migraine development. Some people tend to be awakened early in the morning with a headache, the most common time for migraine to develop. Others find

> The time of day, month, or year may have an effect on when migraine develops.

that their migraine starts in the middle of the day and worsens in the evening, often as they are trying to get through work.

Another migraine pattern is the *weekend headache*. Typically, a somewhat stressed worker will not have migraines despite a very active work week. On Saturday morning, however, she wakes up with a severe migraine headache and is further debilitated with nausea and vomiting, ruining most of Saturday. Three possible explanations explain this phenomenon. One is that the let-down or release of stress has allowed the headache that was building up for several days to be expressed. A second explanation could be oversleeping, because too much sleep may be a trigger for headache. The third explanation is caffeine withdrawal, since the first cup of coffee may come later on Saturdays than during the week. Keeping the weekend schedule similar to weekdays, especially waking hours and caffeine intake, may help.

Some patients have seasonal headaches—for example, migraine that occurs only in winter or spring. No one knows what causes the migraine to appear only at certain times of the year. The causes of seasonal headache patterns vary. It could be that a particular stress, such as school, is only present at that particular time of year; it could be that allergies are triggered; or there could be some as yet unexplained link between the part of the brain that recognizes seasonal changes and the generator of the migraine headache. For example, normal biorhythms fluctuate due to the amount of daily sunlight, triggering headache.

Migraine Triggers

Common migraine triggers include menstruation, stress, relaxation after stress, fatigue, too much or too little sleep, skipping a meal, weather changes, high humidity, high altitude, exposure to glare or flickering lights, loud noises, perfumes or chemical fumes, postural changes, physical activity, or coughing. Food triggers occur in many adult migraineurs and most often include alcoholic beverages (especially red wine), citrus fruits, and foods containing monosodium glutamate, nitrates, and aspartate. Some believe that the desire to eat chocolate is part of the prodrome (anticipation) of migraine. Caffeine use and caffeine withdrawal may also trigger a migraine headache.

CHRONIC MIGRAINE

When migraines become increasingly frequent, occurring on a daily or near-daily basis, they are referred to as *chronic* or *transformed* migraine. By definition, the headaches of chronic migraine occur more than 15 days a month. They need not occur every single day. Often, the less severe of these headaches resemble tension-type headache, with migrainous features becoming increasingly evident as the headache becomes more severe.

Chronic migraine evolves as it develops. It may go through a number of stages: at first, you may only suffer an occasional migraine; then they become more frequent. The next stage is called *early chronic daily headache* (the headaches are not daily, but they occur more often than 15 days a month). Next, the headache is daily, but there is some time when you are headache-free. The final stage is continuous, never-ending headache.

Chronic migraine is surprisingly common. Approximately 1.5 to 2 percent of the population experiences chronic migraine. It is the most common type of headache seen in headache clinics.

Chronic migraine has a much more profound effect on quality of life than episodic migraine. Many chronic migraine sufferers are unable to work at a regular job and their relationships with family, friends, and

> Chronic migraine has a much more profound effect on quality of life than episodic migraine.

colleagues are profoundly affected. Not surprisingly, people who have chronic migraine are more likely to be depressed than those who have episodic migraine.

Chronic migraine frequently develops in conjunction with the overuse of pain or acute migraine medicine. This disorder has been called *rebound* headache or *analgesic overuse* headache.

John had suffered from episodic migraine for some time. The headaches only occurred four or five times a month, but were so severe that he missed work. His doctor prescribed Percocet®. This worked for him, and he was able to function so well that he received a promotion. With the increased responsibility came increased stress, and he noticed that the Percocet® was no longer working as well. Sometimes he had to take two. He also noticed that his prescription needed to be refilled more often. Was he really taking that much more medicine? He called his doctor, who prescribed Fiorinal® with codeine for the headaches that Percocet® couldn't handle. This worked for a while, but it, too, began to be less effective. Soon he was taking some sort of headache medicine almost every day and often more than once a day.

John suffers from rebound headache, which occurs when an occasional headache develops into a daily, or almost daily headache, and the medication that used to work no longer does so. A medical or psychological stressor might trigger a bout of more frequent migraines. Needing to function, the patient takes headache medicine, but the need for medicine increases, and so does the frequency of use. Eventually, higher doses of medicine and then more potent types of medicine become necessary.

Analgesic overuse or rebound can occur with nonprescription products, such as acetaminophen (Tylenol®); aspirin; aspirin combinations (Excedrin®); short-acting, nonsteroidal agents, such as ibuprofen or Motrin®; and almost any acute prescription medicine. People who use medicine for five or six days, such as medications for bad menstrual migraine, but then do not use medicine for weeks or longer do not need to be concerned about rebound.

Linda developed occasional migraines at age 13 and by age 18 had frequent tension-type headaches and monthly migraines. By the age of 25, she was taking Tylenol® half the days of the month. By age 30, she was taking Excedrin® three-quarters of the month. Now 35, she takes four to six Excedrin® almost every day, Imitrex® four days a week, and Fioricet® 10 days a month. She misses three days of work a month and is there "in body but not in spirit" four or five days a month. She does much of the parenting of her two children while lying on the couch. She has seen two neurologists for her migraines and is dissatisfied with the care she receives.

Linda has a moderately severe case of chronic migraine with rebound. Her problem can best be understood by looking at how her problem evolved over decades, *not* by focusing on her most severe attacks. She must first get out of rebound, find an appropriate preventive medicine, and then make lifestyle changes that promote good headache control. Treatment will not be easy, but her prognosis is good.

Joseph had migraine without aura at age six, and then in his teens and 20s. They occurred several times a month. In his 30s, he took aspirin every day "just to prevent the headaches from getting bad." In his late 30s, he was involved in a car accident, had some financial stress, and had to help manage the affairs of his elderly parents. He soon was taking stronger and stronger narcotics. He obtained these medicines by convincing his doctors that using narcotics was the only way for him to get over each financial or social crisis. When he was diagnosed with rebound, he was able to stay off narcotics for one month, during which time he admits (reluctantly) that he took aspirins almost every day. He concluded that he did not have rebound headache and was able to convince his physicians to continue prescribing narcotic pain medicines. Three months ago, he developed the flu; his headaches got worse and he had to stop working. He now takes six strong narcotic tablets (Percocet®) and 10 aspirins a day. He is upset by the diagnosis of rebound headache. Many preventive treatments have failed.

Joseph has severe rebound headache. He is not addicted to narcotic pain medicines, and attempting to treat him as though he were will probably harm him psychologically. His disorder has progressed in part because well-meaning doctors kept him going by increasing the dosage and potency of his pain medicines until the system finally broke. Although he temporarily stopped taking narcotics, he was never effectively "detoxified."

Joseph will need to be hospitalized to get off all pain medicines. Intravenous dihydroergotamine will make this less horrible than he suspects it will be. After hospitalization, however, his significant headaches will return. If Joseph can stay out of rebound and find an effective preventive, over time he is likely to return to normal function.

The most effective tool to determine whether you are rebounding is to keep a headache calendar. You should note the time and severity of

> The most effective tool to determine whether you are rebounding is to keep a headache calendar.

your migraines on the calendar, what you took or did for them, and how well it worked. Examining the calendar, you should look for (1) a pattern of worsening or more frequent headaches, particularly severe headaches, within hours or days of discontinuing acute migraine medicines; (2) an increase in the amount of medication you are taking; or (3) preventive medicines or nonmedical treatments that previously worked well for you and no longer do so.

Rebound may not have all these features. For example, a person who uses six acetaminophen tablets a day might discontinue pain medicines for three months and still have daily headaches as severe as when she was using the drug. Such a person should not resume taking pain medications with the thought that she was never rebounding in the first place. Unless the treatment plan is changed, the headaches will probably not go away. This means changing both the preventive medicines and the nondrug treatment plan. However, the preventive plan will never work well if the individual continues to overuse acetaminophen. In others words, the headaches only meet the third criteria of rebound listed above.

CHAPTER 7

Treating Migraine with Medication

THIS CHAPTER DISCUSSES the various types of medications used by physicians to prevent and control migraine.

MEDICATION FOR ACUTE MIGRAINE

Medication for acute migraine acts to stop headache pain once it has begun and prevents its progression. There are two kinds of medication for acute migraine: specific and nonspecific. Specific treatments are for headache

> Medication for acute migraine acts to stop headache pain once it has begun and prevents its progression.

pain only. Nonspecific medications work on other kinds of pain as well as head pain—for example, they work on nausea as well as migraine, or they work in other painful or inflammatory conditions (see Table 7-1).

Selecting a Treatment for Acute Migraine

Many treatment options for acute migraine are available; some are non-prescription and others require a prescription. How does the migraineur

> Many treatment options for acute migraine are available; some are nonprescription and others require a prescription.

Table 7-1 Specific and Nonspecific Acute Migraine Medication

Specific	Nonspecific
Ergotamine	Acetaminophen
Cafergot®	Tylenol®
Ergot	Aspirin
Dihydroergotamine	Combinations of above with or without caffeine
Migranal®	Caffeine–Excedrin®
Triptans	Aspirin-free Excedrin®
Almotriptan–Axert®	Combination with isometheptene
Eletriptan–Relpax®	Midrin®
Frovatriptan–Frova®	Nonsteroidal anti-inflammatory drugs (NSAIDs)
Naratriptan–Amerge®	Ibuprofen–Motrin®, Advil®
Rizatriptan–Maxalt®	Orudis KT®
Sumatriptan–Imitrex®	Naproxen–Aleve®
Zolmitriptan–Zomig®	Many prescription NSAIDs
	Butalbital
	Butalbital–Fiorinal®/Fioricet®/Esgic®
	Opioids
	Codeine–Tylenol®#3, #4
	Propoxyphene–Darvon®
	Hydroxycodene–Vicodin®
	Oxycodone–Percocet®
	Morphine
	Oxymorphone–Numorphan®
	Hydroxymorphine–Dilaudid®
	Butorphanol–Stadol®
	Other pain medications
	Tramadol–Ultram®/Ultracet®
	Nausea Medicine/Neuroleptics
	Prochlorperazine–Compazine®
	Promethazine–Phenergan®
	Steroids
	Prednisone–Deltasone®, Prednicot®
	Dexamethasone–Decadron®
	Methylprednisolone–Medrol®

select the best nonprescription medicine, and how does the physician select the most appropriate prescriptive treatment?

Treatment responses are highly individualized. A "weaker" treatment may work better for an individual with an apparently severe headache. Overall, acetaminophen is the weakest medication, but it has the least potential for stomach or kidney damage. Ibuprofen and aspirin/acetaminophen/caffeine combinations appear to be stronger and work faster, but they have a higher risk of analgesic rebound. Naproxen is a bit slower than some of the other nonprescription treatments, but it has a very low risk of analgesic overuse.

By the time a person sees the doctor, it is likely he will have tried several nonprescription headache medicines. The physician should not waste time with low-potency, ineffective treatments. Several factors are important in selecting a drug:

- Whether the migraineur has severe nausea or vomiting
- The drug's risk of rebound
- The headache's speed of onset
- The headache's ultimate severity
- The headache's duration
- How the person responded to past treatments
- Risk factors for complications from a particular medicine

Recently an important study was conducted to help doctors determine what strategy to use in selecting treatments for their acute migraine patients. It compared two strategies of care: *sequential care* within or between attacks (step care)—in which the doctor selected cheaper, less effective, nonspecific treatments and prescribed the more expensive, more specific medicine only if the nonspecific one failed—and *stratified care*, wherein the doctor selected a specific treatment for a more severe headache. Stratified care, in which specific treatment was used from the outset, led to better outcomes than sequential care.

Simple and Combination Analgesics and NSAIDs

The authors recommend simple analgesics for people with mild to moderate headaches. Many people find headache relief with a simple analgesic, such as aspirin or acetaminophen (Tylenol®), either alone or in combination with caffeine, a well-established analgesic adjuvant. Acetaminophen's efficacy in acute migraine treatment has now been established. The danger of *Reye's Syndrome* makes acetaminophen preferable to aspirin for children younger than 15 who have headaches. Butalbital combination products are useful where available, but medication overuse is an issue. If you are nauseated, your doctor will prescribe *antinausea* medication. Physicians often try naproxen sodium first, but use a range of nonsteroidal anti-inflammatory drugs (NSAIDs), often in combination with an antiemetic (a medication that prevents nausea). Ibuprofen in nonprescription doses is effective, although acetaminophen plus aspirin with caffeine is more effective than ibuprofen. Acetaminophen is another alternative to aspirin or the other NSAIDs for people who have gastritis or a bleeding disorder that precludes taking aspirin and NSAIDs.

Barbiturate-containing medicines, such as Fiorinal®, Fioricet®, and Esgic®, are widely used for migraine. However, because of concerns about medication-overuse headache, they should be used cautiously, and people taking these medications need to be carefully monitored. In fact, these medicines have been removed from the market in many European countries. They may be very useful as back-up medications when other migraine medications fail. One or two tablets or capsules for an individual attack are usually recommended, with a maximum of six per attack. The most frequent adverse reactions are drowsiness and dizziness. Drug use should be limited to no more than two days per week.

If *nonopioid* medications do not provide adequate pain relief, physicians use codeine in combination with simple medications. They also use, in certain circumstances, more potent *opioid* analgesics, such as propoxyphene (Darvon®), butorphanol (Stadol NS®), meperidine (Demerol®), morphine, hydromorphone (Dilaudid®), and oxycodone (Percocet® and Lorcet®), alone and in combination with simple analgesics. Because medication overuse and rebound headache pose a threat with opioid use, they are most appropriate when severe headaches are relatively infrequent. Butorphanol clearly causes rebound headache and medication overuse syndromes. Opioids should not be used more than two days a week, on average. Physicians sometimes use opioids or barbiturate-containing medications more regularly for women with intractable menstrual migraine because the risk of overuse is less, since the headache improves when the menses is over. These drugs are also especially helpful for people who either do not respond to simple analgesics or cannot take ergots or sumatriptan. Pregnant women can use codeine or meperidine (Demerol®), with caution. Opioids are also useful for people who awaken in the middle of the night with a headache. Sedation, while in some circumstances an undesirable side effect, may help the person go back to sleep and awaken headache-free in the morning.

Nausea Medicines and Neuroleptics

Nausea and vomiting can be as disabling as a headache itself. Nausea medicines are closely related to *neuroleptics* (antipsychotic drugs) and many are effective for headache, even if there is no nausea. Delayed gastric empty-

> Nausea and vomiting can be as disabling as a
> headache itself.

ing decreases the effectiveness of oral medication. Metoclopramide (Reglan®) is a nausea medicine that also stimulates normal gastric emptying. Promethazine (Phenergan®) suppositories or ondansetron (Zofran®) can be used by people who cannot tolerate metoclopramide because of side effects. Doctors use antinausea medicines—chlorpromazine (Thorazine®), droperidol, and prochlorperazine (Compazine®)—intravenously, intramuscularly, and by suppository for nausea, vomiting, and pain. Compazine® suppositories are used as a primary treatment for headache and nausea and also as a rescue medication. Giving Compazine® intravenously or intramuscularly can be a therapeutic choice for treating migraine in the physician's office or hospital emergency room. Thorazine® can be administered intravenously, intramuscularly, or as a suppository. It is used in tablet form for a migraine crisis at home to help relieve pain and allow the person to rest.

Droperidol is safe and effective in treating *status migrainosus* (a migraine attack that lasts longer than 72 hours) and migraine that is refractory to treatment. Side effects include sedation and jitteriness, which can be treated with diphenhydramine or benzotropine. A heart rhythm abnormality can occur after using droperidol if a person has a "long QT" abnormality on EKG or if she is taking other medicine that can prolong the QT. QT is a measure of the heart's ability to conduct electrical impulses. A long QT is an abnormality wherein a portion of the heart's electrical activity cycle is prolonged.

Corticosteroids

Corticosteroids, such as prednisone, hydrocortisone, steroids, and dexamethasone (Decadron®), are effective headache treatments. How they work in migraine is uncertain. They can be given intravenously or by mouth, sometimes in tapering doses over a few days. Limiting their use to 3 to 5 days or 3 to 10 consecutive days per month limits the risk of any long-term complications.

Ergotamine and Dihydroergotamine

Physicians sometimes use ergotamine (Cafergot®) to treat a moderate to severe migraine if analgesics do not provide satisfactory headache relief or if they produce significant side effects and cost is a factor. However, with time and experience, the *triptans* are preferred to ergots for most people. Some people still respond preferentially to rectal ergotamine (Cafergot® suppositories). People who cannot tolerate ergotamine because of nausea are pretreated with an antiemetic. For individual attacks, migraineurs can take up to six 1 mg tablets or two suppositories over 24 hours, but use should not exceed two dosage days per week. In certain circumstances, these limits may be liberalized—for example, in cluster headache or intractable menstrual migraine.

Dihydroergotamine (DHE) has fewer side effects than ergotamine and can be administered intranasally, intramuscularly, subcutaneously, or intravenously. The nasal spray is not as effective as the other routes of administration, but it is very well tolerated. Doctors limit monthly use to 18 ampules or 12 events. DHE remains useful because it is effective for most people; it is associated with a low headache recurrence rate (less than 20 percent); and it is less likely than ergotamine to exacerbate nausea or produce rebound headache.

Women who are attempting to become pregnant and people with uncontrolled hypertension, sepsis, kidney or liver failure, and coronary, cerebral, or peripheral vascular disease should avoid ergotamine and DHE. Nausea is a common side effect of ergotamine, but it is less common with DHE, unless it is given intravenously. Other side effects include dizziness, *paresthesias* (numbness and tingling), abdominal cramps, and chest tightness. Rare unpredictable arterial and coronary vasospasm can also occur. Your doctor may recommend an electrocardiogram before your first dose of DHE, particularly if there are any cardiac risk factors, including those older than 40 years.

Triptans (Selective 5-HT1 Agonists)

Sumatriptan

The first marketed selective serotonin agonist (triptan) was sumatriptan, followed by zolmitriptan (Zomig®), naratriptan (Amerge®), rizatriptan (Maxalt®), almotriptan (Axert®), frovatriptan (Frova®), and eletriptan (Relpax®). Sumatriptan is the most extensively studied agent in the history of migraine, with over nine million individual people and over 400 million attacks treated as of December 2001, but the use of other triptans is increasing. All triptans relieve headache pain, nausea, photophobia, and phonophobia and restore the person's ability to function normally.

Although 80 percent of migraineurs get pain relief from an initial subcutaneous dose of sumatriptan and approximately 60 percent get relief with most oral triptans, headache recurs in about one-third of them. Recurrences are most likely in people with long-duration headaches. Recurrences respond well to a second dose of a triptan or to simple and combination analgesics.

None of the triptans should be used by people who have diseased heart arteries, *Prinzmetal's angina*, uncontrolled hypertension, *vertebrobasilar* migraine, or who are at high risk for these conditions. Common side effects include pain at injection sites, tingling, flushing, burning, and warm or hot sensations. Dizziness, heaviness, neck pain, fatigue, and mood changes also can occur. These side effects generally abate within 45 minutes. Chest pressure that has nothing to do with heart trouble occurs in approximately 4 percent of those with migraines. When migraineurs are over the age of 40 years or have risk factors for heart disease, physicians obtain an EKG before using sumatriptan. Adverse events—most commonly malaise/fatigue, dizziness/vertigo, weakness, and nausea—are generally more frequent (and in some cases significantly more frequent) with the oral triptans than with *placebo*. Doctors sometimes give the first dose of sumatriptan in the office at a time when the patient does not have a headache.

Seven triptans are currently available. They are safe for people who do not have cardiovascular risk factors, and they are an effective first-line therapy for people who have a moderate to severe migraine headache, or for whom analgesics have failed to provide adequate relief.

Headache severity, rapidity of onset, and duration are important factors when deciding which triptan should be used. When the headache intensifies rapidly (in less than 30 minutes), or nausea and vomiting are early and severe associated symptoms, nonoral administration is appropriate. Subcutaneous sumatriptan is the fastest and most effective. Sumatriptan or zolmitriptan nasal spray may provide relief faster than oral triptans, but sumatriptan nasal spray is often associated with a disagreeable taste.

The oral formulations can be divided into two classes:

- Almotriptan, eletriptan, rizatriptan, sumatriptan, and zolmitriptan have the highest two-hour efficacy; they can provide headache relief within 30 to 60 minutes; and they would be the first choice when migraineurs require efficacy and speedy relief and do not have multiple recurrences.
- Frovatriptan and naratriptan have lower two-hour efficacy, but fewer side effects (as does almotriptan). Almotriptan, frovatriptan, and naratriptan are the best choices for those who are prone to side effects.

All triptans have the same contraindications and safety concerns. None is safer than another. However, the response to triptans is often idiosyncratic. One triptan may work for one person and cause no side effects, and a different triptan may work for another person. The triptan of choice is the one that restores the migraineur's ability to function by swiftly and consistently relieving pain and associated symptoms with minimum side effects and without recurrence of symptoms.

Early intervention prevents escalation and may increase efficacy. Triptans can prevent the development of *cutaneous allodynia* (nonpainful stimuli, such as combing your hair becomes painful) which is important, because once allodynia has been present for more than one hour, triptans are much less effective. Treat at least two attacks with a new medication before deciding that the medication is ineffective. It may be necessary for your doctor to change the dose, formulation, or route of administration, or add an adjuvant (for example, an antinausea medicine). When the response is inadequate, the headache recurs, or side effects are bothersome, a medication change may be needed. All treatments occasionally fail and, therefore, rescue medications, such as opioids, neuroleptics, and corticosteroids, may be needed. They provide relief, but often limit function due to sedation or other side effects.

Treat Early or Late

It is clear that early treatment gets rid of migraine more quickly and more completely than if treatment is delayed. Early treatment also

> It is clear that early treatment gets rid of migraine more quickly and more completely than if treatment is delayed.

reduces the number of pills needed to treat each attack, but be careful—it may increase the risk of overuse and chronic daily headache in people with frequent migraine.

If you are likely to treat four or fewer headaches a month, treat as early as possible. The gray zone is the 5 to 8 headache days per month and, in this case, some limits may need to be set for early treatments. You may not be able to treat early most of the time if you need to treat more than eight days a month. In the last two cases, you may benefit from really studying your headaches to determine what symptoms predict a headache that will become severe. Discussing early versus late treatment with your doctor may help you get the best control of individual attacks without getting into rebound.

PREVENTIVE TREATMENT

Preventive medications are taken on a daily basis (usually for over a month), whether or not headache is present, in order to reduce attack

> Preventive medications are taken on a daily basis (usually for over a month), whether or not headache is present, in order to reduce attack frequency, duration, or severity.

frequency, duration, or severity. Preventive treatment can be preemptive, short-term, or long-term.

Preemptive treatment is used when there is a known headache trigger, such as exercise or sexual activity, or a clear prodrome or aura symptom indicating impending headache. Migraineurs are instructed to treat the headache before it begins, with a single dose of a preemptive agent. For example, single doses of indomethacin 25 or 50 mg can be given 1 to 2 hours prior to exercise to prevent exercise-induced migraine.

Short-term prevention (*mini-prophylaxis*) is used when there is an expectation of limited exposure to a provoking factor, such as menstruation or ascent to a high altitude. Treatment is taken for several days during the period of increased headache risk. Examples of this include using NSAIDs or frovatriptan daily for one week before the expected onset of menstruation for menstrual migraine.

Recommendations for long-term migraine prevention often focus on the number of attacks that occur each month, but this should not be the only factor considered. Circumstances that warrant ongoing preventive treatment include:

- Recurring migraine that significantly interferes with the migraineur's daily routine despite acute treatment—for example, two or more attacks a month that produce disability that lasts three or more days, or headache attacks that are infrequent, but produce profound disability.

- Failure of, contraindication to, or troublesome side effects from acute medications.
- Overuse of acute medications.
- Special circumstances, such as *hemiplegic* migraine or attacks, with a risk of permanent neurologic injury.
- Very frequent headaches (more than two a week), with the concomitant risk of rebound headache development.
- Preference: the desire to have as few acute attacks as possible.

Preventive medications should be avoided during pregnancy unless severe pain or disability creates benefits from medication that overshadow the risks. The major medication groups for preventive migraine treatment include beta-adrenergic blockers, antidepressants, calcium channel antagonists, serotonin antagonists, nerve modulators, and NSAIDs. If preventive medication is indicated, the agent should be chosen from one of the major categories, based on side-effect profiles and coexistent or *comorbid* conditions (separate conditions that tend to occur together).

Preventive medication should be started at a low dose and increased slowly until it starts working, side effects develop, or a maximum dose

> Preventive medication should be started at a low dose and increased slowly until it starts working, side effects develop, or a maximum dose is reached.

is reached. Migraineurs frequently require a lower dose of a preventive medication than the same medication taken for other medical problems. While some people respond to lower doses of preventive medications, not all do, and it may be necessary to increase the dose to tolerance before assuming the agent is ineffective.

A full trial of medication may take 2 to 6 months. Medicine often does not start to work until it has been used for four weeks; benefits may continue to increase over three months of therapy. It is not uncommon for someone to be treated with a new preventive medication for 1 to 2 weeks without effect and then prematurely discontinue it, based on the mistaken belief that it is not effective.

To obtain benefit from preventive medication, do not overuse analgesics or ergot derivatives. In addition, oral contraceptives, hormonal replacement therapy, or *vasodilating* drugs, such as nifedipine or nitroglycerin, may interfere with preventive drugs.

Migraine headaches may improve with time independent of treatment, and if the headaches are well-controlled, slow drug withdrawal can be undertaken. Many people experience continued relief after discontinuing the medication or may not need to resume drug treatment. Dose reduction may provide continuous benefit with fewer side effects.

A woman of childbearing potential should be on adequate contraception before starting migraine medication. However, some women who are pregnant, or who are attempting to become pregnant, may still require preventive medications. If this is absolutely necessary, the patient needs to work with her doctor to evaluate the potential risks and pick the medication with the fewest potential adverse effects on the fetus.

PREVENTIVE MEDICATIONS

Beta-Blockers

Propranolol (Inderal®), metoprolol (Toprol®), timolol (Blocadren®), nadolol (Corgard®), and atenolol (Tenormin®) are all effective beta-blockers. Doctors often use timolol or propranolol because they have the strongest evidence of effectiveness. Since beta-blockers can produce behavioral side effects, such as drowsiness, fatigue, lethargy, sleep disorders, nightmares, depression, memory disturbance, and hallucinations, doctors avoid prescribing them when migraineurs have depression or low energy. Decreased exercise tolerance limits their use by athletes. Less common side effects include impotence, *orthostatic hypotension* (abnormal drop in blood pressure upon standing), significant *bradycardia* (slow heart rate), and aggravation of muscle disease. Physicians find beta-blockers especially useful for people with *angina* or hypertension.

They are relatively contraindicated for those with congestive heart failure, asthma, Raynaud's disease, and insulin-dependent diabetes.

Antidepressants

The currently available antidepressants used in migraine treatment consist of a number of different classes with different mechanisms of action: nonselective tricyclic antidepressants (TCAs), selective serotonin reuptake inhibitors (SSRIs), and selective serotonin and *norepinephrine* reuptake inhibitors (SNRIs).

The TCAs are most commonly used for migraine and tension-type headache prevention. The only one that has been absolutely proven effective is amitriptyline (Elavil®), but nortriptyline (Pamelor®) and protriptyline (Vivactil®) are often used, based largely on clinical experience and uncontrolled reports. Physicians often use TCAs for people who have trouble sleeping, and SSRIs, such as fluoxetine, paroxetine, and sertraline, to treat co-existent depression, based on their favorable side-effect profiles, not their established efficacy. Fluoxetine (Prozac®) is of proven value in chronic daily headache and may work for migraine.

Side effects from TCAs are common, usually dry mouth and sedation. The drugs also cause increased appetite and weight gain; cardiac toxicity and low blood pressure occur occasionally. Sexual dysfunction, which is treatable, is not uncommon with the use of SSRIs.

Calcium Channel Blockers

Calcium channel blockers are a type of blood pressure medicine often used to control migraines. Of the calcium channel blockers available in the USA, verapamil (Calan®) is the most widely used and has the best evidence to support its use. Verapamil is especially useful for people who have high blood pressure or contraindications—such as asthma and Raynaud's disease—to beta-blockers. Physicians also use verapamil for people who have *migrainous infarction* or migraine with prolonged aura. Nifedipine is also used occasionally. Low blood pressure is a less common side effect with calcium channel blockers than with beta-blockers. Constipation and swelling of the legs may occur.

Neuromodulating Drugs

Neuromodulating drugs (NMDs) (anti-epileptic drugs) are increasingly recommended for migraine prevention because they have proven to be effective. Divalproex sodium was the first NMD proven to effectively control migraines. It is available in an extended release form, which has side effects similar to placebo. The most frequent side effects are nausea, hair loss, tremor, fatigue, upset stomach, sleepiness, and weight gain. Very rarely liver problems and occasionally pancreatitis can develop. Before starting an individual on Depakote®, doctors check liver function, and if it is normal they do not routinely repeat liver function tests.

For many people, divalproex is effective at a low dose of 500 to 1000 mg per day, as opposed to the 2000 to 5000 mg per day dose that people with epilepsy may require. It can be given as an extended release preparation at bedtime.

Gabapentin (Neurontin®) is effective in reducing the frequency of migraine attacks, but only at a higher dose. The most common adverse events are dizziness, giddiness, and drowsiness.

Topiramate is the newest drug proven effective in controlling migraines. Topiramate should be started at a dose of 25mg/day at bedtime and increased weekly until the target dose of 100 mg/day in two divided doses is reached. Some individuals may need a higher dose. Topiramate side effects include tingling, loss of appetite, diarrhea, weight loss, concentration and memory problems. These side effects usually go away when the medication is discontinued. Starting at a low dose and increasing the dose slowly can often reduce side effects.

Serotonin Antagonists

Methysergide (Sansert®) is effective in preventing migraine. Side effects include transient muscle aching, muscle pain, abdominal pain, nausea, weight gain, and hallucinations. Frightening hallucinations can occur after the first dose. The manufacturer has discontinued production of methysergide, and some physicians are now using methergine instead of methysergide (the body converts methysergide to methergine anyway). The major complication of methysergide and methergine is the rare (1 in 2,500) development of fibrosis around the kidneys, in the heart valves, or around the heart or lungs. A medication-free interval of four weeks following each six-month course of continuous treatment is recommended to prevent this complication.

Neurotoxins

The latest buzz in headache circles concerns Botox® (*botulinum toxin A*). Botox® is a *neurotoxin* that weakens muscles by blocking the release of acetylcholine, a substance that transmits messages to the muscles. For the last 20 years, Botox® has been used to treat a variety of disorders characterized by inappropriate and involuntary muscle contraction. It is effective and has been approved for treating squinting (*blepharospasm*), facial spasm, and wrinkles. It has also been safely used for spasticity, tremor, and abnormal sweating. The effects of treatment last 3 to 6 months.

The fact that Botox® can be an effective headache treatment was discovered by serendipity—patients told their doctors that their headaches improved when they were given Botox® to treat other conditions. This led to further investigation of its effectiveness for migraine and tension-type headaches, as well as other painful conditions.

The reason Botox® inhibits pain is not known and this is under investigation. However, the injectable drug does seem to inhibit the pain associated with migraine and other types of headache. The authors' medical center conducted and published the results of the first clinical trial of Botox® for migraine, which showed at the end of the three-month trial that participants had a significant reduction in attacks. Most of the people in this study had no side effects. However, a few of them did report transient minor side effects, including eyelid droop, double vision, and injection-site weakness. Botox® may be an effective and well-tolerated therapy for the prevention of migraine and other headache disorders, including tension-type headache and the headache of cervical *dystonia* (an involuntary posture or movement). Its effects are long-lasting—they may last over four months—and the drug has no systemic or serious side effects.

SPECIAL CIRCUMSTANCES

Menstrual Migraine

Many women get migraine and menstrual cramps with their period. First, consider the use of a NSAID for this problem, such as ibuprofen or naproxen, when the pain occurs or even on a daily basis (*miniprophylaxis*). The triptans are very effective for the acute treatment of menstrual migraine—they can also be used for miniprophylaxis. Many obstetricians/gynecologists have their patients take oral contraceptives for three months in a row without the pill-free (or placebo) week. This results in fewer menstrual periods and less headache. The headaches may return when the oral contraceptives are stopped.

Exercise Headache

Some individuals get headache from exercise. Warm up slowly. Take a NSAID, such as ibuprofen or naproxen, before exercise and stay well-hydrated.

> Some individuals get headache from exercise. Warm up slowly.

Hospitalization for Headache

Chronic migraine with severe disability and uncontrolled migraine status may warrant hospitalization to break the cycle of pain and restore the migraineur to normal function. Criteria for hospitalization include:

- Failure of multiple aggressive outpatient interventions, including outpatient intravenous treatment.
- Failure to control overuse of pain medicines, despite aggressive outpatient plan and education.
- Overuse of a large amount of barbiturates (Fiorinal® or Esgic®) or opioids (codeine, Oxycodene®, or Percocet®).

- Severe desperation, up to and including risk of suicide.
- Impending loss of job or withdrawal from school unless migraine is rapidly controlled.

Headache centers may schedule hospitalizations in order to make resources and expertise available.

CHAPTER 8

Alternative Therapies
for Migraine

S OME MIGRAINEURS TRY nondrug or behavioral treatment to manage
their headaches before resorting to drug or physical therapy. Others
treat their headaches concurrently with drug and behavioral therapies.
Still others rely strictly on drugs. Because behavioral treatments do not
increase headaches, and often help to decrease them, it is generally fool-
ish to ignore these low-cost and effective treatment methods.

Managing headache pain, particularly the pain of chronic headache,
often goes beyond simply popping a pill. Medication can do a great deal

> Managing headache pain, particularly the
> pain of chronic headache, often goes beyond
> simply popping a pill.

toward relieving pain, but headache sufferers, particularly those plagued
with a chronic form of headache, can usually benefit from an overall
lifestyle plan incorporating alternative therapies. Along with appropriate
medication, a properly balanced lifestyle, including a healthy diet, regular sleeping hours, and some degree of exercise, will almost always
reduce the frequency and severity of headaches.

A headache sufferer needs a carefully designed plan, and to assist
you and your doctor in creating a plan, we have divided treatment four
ways (see diagram on next page).

People with a mild or infrequent headache problem need only a
treatment that fits into the acute drug treatment box. If the headache
problem is more severe or difficult to manage, more types of treatment

Drug	Acute	Preventive
Nondrug	Body	Mind

should be used. Anyone with frequent, difficult-to-manage headaches needs at least one treatment of each type.

This chapter offers headache sufferers an overview of the different therapies available and the potential advantages and disadvantages associated with each. For simplification purposes, we will use the classifications of dietary, physical, and behavioral therapies.

DIETARY SUPPLEMENTS

Dietary supplements lie somewhere between traditional and nontraditional headache therapies. They are closest to traditional preventive

> Dietary supplements lie somewhere between traditional and nontraditional headache therapies.

medications in the way they are administered and the way they act. Most are vitamin, herbal, or botanical preparations.

Vitamins

Several vitamin supplements have been studied and found to be helpful in managing headache. Riboflavin (vitamin B2), at a dose of 400 mg per day, reduces the frequency of headache attacks and the number of headache days. It also improves the production of ATP, the principal energy-storing molecule. Magnesium has been effective in some studies and ineffective in others, but when administered intravenously, it has shown possibilities in treating acute attacks.

Coenzyme Q is a nutritional supplement that has recently been shown to reduce the frequency of migraine attacks. Like B2, it improves the cell's energy production. Two studies of coenzyme Q have been performed: one using a dose of 150 mg twice a day, and a smaller one using 150 mg once a day. While the evidence is strongest for twice a day dosing, coenzyme Q is a bit more expensive than B2 or magnesium and the twice a day dose may be too expensive for some.

Hydroxycobalamine—a form of vitamin B12—also seems promising. It is a nitric oxide scavenger, which is thought to be involved in headache production. It has been shown to be effective in a significant number of cases when taken intranasally, but it will take more studies to confirm this.

Pyridoxine (vitamin B6) is used as supportive treatment for people with *histamine* intolerance, believed to be involved in some cases of food- and wine-induced chronic headaches. People with this sensitivity should follow a diet that does not promote a histamine reaction. They should also avoid alcohol and diamine-oxidase blocking drugs. The recommended dose of vitamin B6 is 100 to 150 mg per day; higher doses have proven toxic in some individuals. Moreover, pyridoxine can raise serotonin levels, possibly reversing the lack of this neurotransmitter in migraineurs.

One preliminary clinical trial showed that long-term use of S-adenosylmethionine (SAM-e) offered possible benefits for migraine treatment by possibly affecting serotonin production.

Vitamin A is not a treatment for migraine, but it is important to mention that overuse of this supplement has been shown to cause *pseudotumor cerebri*, which can be associated with severe chronic headaches and visual disturbances.

Vitamins and botanicals can be potentially harmful, especially when the dose is too high. Therefore, high doses of vitamins should not be randomly used. A balanced diet containing all the necessary nutrients is the best approach.

Herb and Botanical Treatments

Herbs and botanicals not only treat acute pain, but they may relax and balance the body for longer-lasting benefits.

Herbs and botanicals not only treat acute pain, but they may relax and balance the body for longer-lasting benefits.

The most commonly used therapies in this class are:

- Inhalation using melissa, peppermint, and chamomile.
- Massage with lavender, peppermint, anise, basil, and eucalyptus.
- Warm baths with eucalyptus, wintergreen, and peppermint.
- Compresses of peppermint, ginger and marjoram, and vinegar.
- Other recommended treatments include warm salt packs, herbal footbaths, icy footbaths, cold sitz baths, cold and then hot wrist baths, and tight headbands.

In one German study, the combination of peppermint oil and eucalyptus oil as a topical preparation increased cognitive performance and had a muscle-relaxing and mental-relaxing effect, but it had little influence on pain. A significant positive effect on pain was produced by a combination of peppermint oil and ethanol.

Feverfew (*Tanacetum parthenium*), also known as featherfew and bachelor's buttons, is native to southwestern Europe and has been used to treat disorders often controlled by aspirin. Studies show conflicting evidence of its effectiveness for headaches, and feverfew has been thought to contribute to rebound. This substance should not be used with warfarin, as it may increase bleeding times.

An extract of butterbur root (petasites/Petadolex®) has been tested as a migraine preventive, with successful results and virtually no side effects. These studies need to be compared with future trials for confirmed evidence of the root's effectiveness. No studies demonstrate that ginger (*Zingiber officinale*) works in headache, although the Ayurvedic and Tibb systems of medicine propose it as an abortive and preventive treatment option. The bark of the stately white willow tree (*Salix alba*) has been used in China for centuries because of its ability to relieve pain and lower fever. Ingested as tea or capsules, it has an active ingredient related to aspirin.

Passionflower, skullcap, and hops are sometimes included in preparations for headache, but there have been no clinical trials showing significant benefits. Cannabis (marijuana) was a preferred migraine treatment from 1842 until 1942. The first evidence of its use goes back to the year 5000 B.C., with the first documented use for headache seen in the year 300 B.C. The authors have treated headache sufferers for a number of years and have not seen anyone who reports sustained benefit from using this substance for headache. There have also been reports of marijuana being associated with increased headache. One study suggested that migraine usually precedes marijuana use and tension-type headache usually develops after chronic use. The potentially intoxicating effect, possible long-term harm with frequent use, and societal stigmatization associated with this herb are likely to restrict its medicinal use for headache.

High doses of most vitamins, minerals, or botanicals are not advised during pregnancy (see Table 8-1). However, the use of folate is strongly urged for all pregnant women and, in fact, is recommended for all women of child-bearing potential. The use of oral magnesium is also acceptable for pregnant women, because blood levels do not rise above normal in persons who do not have kidney failure.

Physical Treatments

Physical Therapy

Physical therapy is used to strengthen neck muscles, improve mobility, and correct poor posture. Physical therapy can include the use of moist heating pads, which are applied to ease pain and improve mobility, ultrasound, and massage for short-term pain relief, as well as strengthening and stretching exercises for long-term prevention of pain. Many people who have headaches experience a great deal of muscle tightness

> Physical therapy is used to strengthen neck muscles, improve mobility, and correct poor posture.

TABLE 8-1 Benefits and Harm of Vitamins, Botanicals, and Herbs

Vitamin/ Botanical	Type of Headache or Related Condition	Evidence of Harm
Butterbur	Migraine–preventive	None
Cannabis	Migraine–tension-type headache	Tension-type headache with chronic use
Cocaine	Headache trigger, cluster No evidence of benefit	Hemorrhages, vasoconstriction
Coenzyme Q	Migraine–preventive	Not known
Ephedra	Energy enhancer, weight loss No evidence of benefit	CNS toxicity (strokes, death)
Feverfew	Migraine–preventive	None
Folic Acid	Migraine–preventive No evidence of benefit	Not known
Ginger	Migraine–possible preventive? No evidence of benefit	Not known
Gingko biloba	Migraine–possible preventive? No evidence of benefit	Not known
Hydroxycobalamine	Migraine–preventive	Not known
Kava kava	Anxiety No evidence of benefit	Liver toxicity
Magnesium	Migraine–preventive	Diarrhea
Passionflower	Sleep disorders? No evidence of benefit	None
Peppermint oil	Migraine–abortive	None
Pueraria root	Migraine–symptomatic No evidence of benefit	Not known
Pyridoxine-B6	Histamine-induced headache	Nerve damage (in high doses)
Riboflavin-B2	Migraine–preventive	Not known
SAM-e	Migraine–preventive	Not known
Tobacco	Headache trigger No evidence of benefit	Multiple adverse health effects
Vitamin A	Migraine? No evidence of benefit	Pseudotumor cerebri, hypercalcemia
Vitamin E	Dapsone-induced headache	Not known
White willow bark	Acute No evidence of benefit	None

in the upper back and neck. Loosening muscle spasms may help to relieve migraine pain. Application of cold is also used when some areas are too tender to massage or stretch. Ice packs or vapo-coolant spray can be used to cool the skin, allowing the therapist to stretch tender muscles without pain.

Cervical manipulation (movement of the neck by a therapist) is sometimes used to treat migraines. Maneuvers include *mobilization*—in which the therapist passively moves a joint or group of joints to the limit of the usual physiologic range of movement and then returns to the starting point—and *manipulation*, during which a thrust is administered after the limit of the usual physiologic range of movement has been attained. This maneuver takes the range slightly beyond the usual, typically with the accompaniment of a "cracking" noise. These manipulations are done to increase the range of motion of the neck; they should always be performed gently. Manipulation carries with it a remote chance of stroke and should only be used as a last resort.

Acupressure and Shiatsu Massage

Acupressure is an Asian method of finger-pressure massage that targets the acupuncture *meridians*, 12 invisible energy channels throughout the body used in traditional eastern medicine. Blockage of energy flow, or *Qi*, is believed to cause pain, and release of blocked energy promotes wellness. Shiatsu is a similar, but less intense finger-pressure massage that targets the same meridians as acupressure.

Acupuncture

Acupuncture is another Asian technique based on the flow of Qi, the life energy force. This is performed by inserting small needles into points along the meridians. Acupuncture is said to mobilize serotonin and norepinephrine, which block pain transmission and produce *endorphins*, the body's own natural pain-relieving chemicals. A number of studies have not shown it to be effective in the treatment of migraine and tension-type headaches, although a recent study showed the benefits of acupuncture to be similar to those of amitriptyline. Many conventional physicians refrain from fully endorsing the use of acupuncture for migraine, and few agree on how effective acupuncture is in treating pain. It is used as a coadjuvant therapy because there is clear individual variability in response and no evidence of harm.

Chiropractic Care

Physicians have differing opinions on the use of chiropractic techniques for the treatment of migraine headaches. Chiropractors use their hands to manipulate the spine in order to maintain a healthy balance. This approach should be avoided if you have, or are at risk of having certain medical conditions, especially stroke, so be sure to discuss this with your chiropractor before receiving treatment. There is evidence that neck manipulation can on rare occasions cause stroke even in healthy people, so you should understand the risks if you choose this form of treatment.

Craniosacral Therapy

Based on a variation of osteopathic medicine, the main principle of craniosacral therapy is to increase the mobility of the bones in and near the head, reduce the pressure on the nerves of the skull, and improve the flow of blood and cerebrospinal fluid. There are no conclusive studies that show the potential benefit of this therapy as a headache treatment, and success appears to be individualized.

Hydrotherapy

Hydrotherapy is traditionally used as an adjunct treatment to massage. It employs hot and cold packs, saunas, steam baths, and whirlpools.

Massage

Massage, either self-administered or given by therapists, is not only used by headache sufferers, but is effective in alleviating many forms of pain.

Some studies show benefits of massage only during the actual therapy. There are also differences in the effectiveness of massage, depending on the type of headache. Nevertheless, massage helps relax muscles, release the tension in tendons and other soft tissues, improve circulation, increase the uptake of oxygen, and stimulate the production of endorphins.

Reflexology (Zone Therapy)

The principles of reflexology are similar to those of acupressure and shiatsu in that areas and points on the hands, feet, head, and ears correspond to other body areas. Applying massage or pressure to specific areas enhances the well-being of the associated organs.

Qijong

Qijong is the skill of working with the "life force" by using movement and meditation to reduce stress, blood pressure, and muscle tension.

Yoga

The word *yoga* comes from the Hindu tradition and means "to yoke, unite, or integrate." This is not just a physical technique, but also a way of life that trains the body, mind, and emotions to unite with the spirit. The benefits of yoga are many, including an increase in blood flow, release of tension, production of endorphins, removal of toxins, and regulation of serotonin.

BEHAVIORAL THERAPIES

Behavioral therapies are useful for headache sufferers who prefer not to use drugs, including those:

- Who have trouble tolerating drugs.
- Who are allergic or have other medical reasons to avoid drugs.
- For whom drugs work poorly.
- Who are pregnant, planning a pregnancy, or nursing.

- Who have a history of excessive use of analgesic or other acute medications.
- Who have a psychological disorder, poor coping skills, or life stresses that aggravate headache problems.

Behavioral treatments are often administered in small groups, allowing the cost of treatment to be reduced. The goals of behavioral therapy include reducing the frequency and severity of headaches, lessening any headache-related disability, lowering reliance on medications—particularly if poorly tolerated or unwanted—and enhancing personal control of headaches.

Behavioral treatments are classified into three broad categories: relaxation training, biofeedback therapy, and cognitive-behavioral or stress-management training. Biofeedback and relaxation therapy also help people manage stress, especially children, pregnant women, and those whose headaches are brought on by stress.

Relaxation Training

The three most widely used types of relaxation training are:

- **Progressive muscle relaxation**—alternately tensing and relaxing selected muscle groups throughout the body.
- **Autogenic training**—promoting a state of deep relaxation by self-instructions of warmth and heaviness.
- **Meditation**—focusing the mind on a sound or silently repeated word, called a mantra, to promote mental calm and relaxation.

Relaxation skills give headache sufferers greater control over the body's responses to headache. Relaxation may also provide an activity break and help the individual gain a sense of mastery or self-control.

> Relaxation skills give headache sufferers greater control over the body's responses to headache.

Hypnotherapy

Hypnotherapy is a state of focused concentration that allows the participant to be highly receptive to suggestion. It was approved by the American Medical Association in 1958 as a therapeutic technique. Hypnotherapy has been shown to produce effects on the body similar to deep relaxation, and a few studies show that it may decrease the frequency and severity of tension-type and migraine headaches.

Relaxation

Relaxation is considered the foundation and by product of many behavioral therapies, and includes techniques that focus on breathing and relaxing muscles. Three types of relaxation trainings are progressive muscle relaxation, autogenic training (using instructions of warmth and heaviness to promote calmness), and meditation. One study showed that after 10 therapy sessions of progressive relaxation training, 96 percent of migraineurs had a reduction in the frequency, duration, and severity of head pain.

Many people are successful at performing self-hypnosis learned from videos or audiotapes. You can lead yourself into deep relaxation using hypnosis. With progressive relaxation, you take yourself through a series of toe-to-head muscle relaxation exercises. You start with your toes, contracting and relaxing individual muscles, and then work your way up, gradually covering all muscle groups. This can be combined with deep breathing. When using visualization or guided imagery, try to picture yourself pain-free in your favorite place to relax, such as the beach, a boat, or by the fireplace in a lodge. Imagery (guided or unguided) and visualization can provide relaxation, as well as directly affect your body. Studies have shown that imagining a place, situation, or thing causes the same changes in the brain as if you were actually experiencing that place, situation, or thing.

The word *meditation* shares the same root as *medicine*, meaning *to cure*. Formal clinical studies of meditation have shown it to be effective in reducing pain, high blood pressure, and heart rate. Changes in chemical blood levels in the body have also been reported. Many forms of

115

meditation exist that help people with headache manage pain and the stress of every-day life. To meditate, sit in a relaxed position, close your eyes, breathe deeply and slowly, and repeat your mantra—if you are using one—or focus on your breath. Deep breathing is often used in conjunction with relaxation techniques.

Biofeedback Training

Biofeedback is the most successfully studied behavioral approach in migraine management. Younger headache sufferers and children show many positive results from using this technique. The technique is so well established as a preventive for migraine that some consider it to be a conventional treatment option (Figure 8-1).

Biofeedback is commonly used in conjunction with relaxation training. The person uses "feedback" about a physiological function to regu-

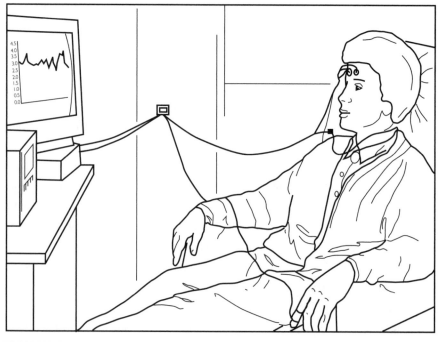

FIGURE 8-1

A patient undergoing electromyographic biofeedback training for frontal muscle relaxation as well as hand temperature biofeedback training.

late the monitored response. For example, thermal (hand warming) feedback monitors skin temperature, whereby you can learn to control the temperature of your hands and feet. *Electromyographic* feedback monitors the electrical activity from the muscles of the scalp, neck, and sometimes the upper body.

Energetic and Spiritual Healing

It has been suggested that the power of these types of therapies lies in the mind of the recipient and the intent of the "healer." To date, there is no scientific evidence supporting the efficacy of these techniques for headache management.

Stress Management Therapy

Managing stress effectively is a useful skill for anyone, but especially for someone with headaches. The way you cope—or do not cope—with everyday stress can bring on a headache, make it worse, or make it last

> The way you cope—or do not cope—with everyday stress can bring on a headache, make it worse, or make it last longer.

longer. It can also increase the disability and distress caused by the headache. Learning to manage stress should be a priority in changing your lifestyle to reduce your headaches.

Stress management focuses on the thoughts and emotional components of headache. Typically, it is administered in conjunction with relaxation training. It emphasizes the role your thoughts play in generating stress and the relationship between stress, your efforts to cope, and your headaches. Stress management techniques will teach you to employ more effective coping strategies.

Some headache sufferers view their headaches as outside their control ("Headaches just happen"), or the result of a personal deficiency ("It must be my fault I have headaches"). Either belief can lead to an attitude of helplessness. This need not be the case. You can monitor your physical reactions, thoughts, and emotional responses to headache-related stresses. Relaxation skills can be used throughout the day. Self-regulation skills can be practiced during headache-free periods before being used to control physiological responses throughout the day or abort an anticipated headache episode. Audiotapes and treatment manuals can repeat and extend what is learned in treatment sessions and homework assignments.

Psychotherapy

Living with the pain and stress of a headache disorder can leave migraineurs feeling helpless, frustrated, anxious, and/or depressed. These emotions can work against them and make the headache condi-

> Several forms of psychotherapy or counseling, such as cognitive therapy, behavioral therapy, and support groups, can be helpful in dealing with the effects of disabling headaches.

tion worse by lowering the ability to tolerate pain and stress. Several forms of psychotherapy or counseling, such as cognitive therapy, behavioral therapy, and support groups, can be helpful in dealing with the effects of disabling headaches. One study showed between 43 and 100 percent improvement of chronic tension-type headache sufferers who were involved in cognitive therapy, as opposed to no improvement in those who were not. Support groups can offer a safe and understanding place to share your struggles and feelings about your headache disorder and help you feel less isolated.

Some Helpful Hints

Try to use simple ways of handling pain, such as walking, neck massage, breathing, and relaxation techniques, before taking pain-relief medication at the first twinge of a headache.

Change what you are doing: If you are washing the dishes when a headache starts, take a walk or read a book. Distraction is effective for many mild headaches.

Stop negative self-talk and replace negative thoughts with positive ones, such as "I'll feel better soon."

Other Primary Headaches and Associated Illnesses

CHAPTER 9

Tension-Type Headache

MOST OF US ARE ALL TOO familiar with tension-type headaches, because at least 80 percent of us will have one at some point in our lives. This type of headache can last from 30 minutes to seven days. The pain may be mild or moderate, pressing or tightening, and usually

> Most of us are all too familiar with tension-type headaches, because at least 80 percent of us will have one at some point in our lives.

occurs on both sides of the head. There is sometimes considerable tenderness of the muscles of the scalp, jaw, and neck. Tension-type headaches are aggravated by the stresses of everyday life and thus may be worse toward the end of the day. This is the headache most people mean when they refer to "just a headache."

John was a 25-year-old salesman who occasionally developed mild pain around his head at the end of the day. He said the headaches felt like a tight band around his head. He never experienced nausea with his headaches, and neither light nor sound bothered him. He would massage his head and take an aspirin, and these measures brought relief.

Tension-type headaches are nondescript and usually not disabling. They often can be treated with just a nonprescription analgesic and relaxation techniques.

Causes of Tension-Type Headache

No one knows what causes tension-type headache. In fact, despite extensive study, even less is known about the cause of tension-type headache than the cause of migraine.

> No one knows what causes tension-type headache.

Some people who have tension-type headaches also have excessive scalp and neck muscle contraction and increased tenderness in these muscles. Psychological studies of people with tension-type headaches do not reveal any consistent findings. However, some studies have shown higher levels of anxiety, depression, and suppressed anger in people with tension-type headaches. In one study, the frequency of headache increased as the frequency of daily annoyances increased. I think most of us would agree with that! However, in the most carefully performed study so far, people who had tension-type headaches did not have more anxiety or other mood problems than people who did not.

When to Seek Help

So when does "just a headache" become a problem serious enough to seek advice from a specialist? Sometimes, people who have tension-type headaches develop what are called *chronic tension-type headaches*. These

> Sometimes, people who have tension-type headaches develop what are called *chronic tension-type headaches.*

headaches are similar to original headaches, usually occur on both sides of the head, and often involve the back of the head and neck.

Chronic tension-type headache is similar to chronic migraine and may be associated with medication overuse or rebound. Almost any pain medicine, including acetaminophen, can cause rebound.

TREATMENT OF TENSION-TYPE HEADACHE

Episodic tension-type headaches are treated with acute medications. If the headaches are more frequent or become chronic, preventive medication is used in conjunction with counseling, stress management, relaxation therapy, and/or biofeedback, as determined by you and your doctor.

Medication

To stop or reduce the severity of the individual attack, the first choice is usually aspirin, acetaminophen (Tylenol®), or ibuprofen, alone or in combination with caffeine, sedatives, or codeine, and nonsteroidal anti-inflammatory drugs (NSAIDs). Some doctors use muscle relaxants as well. The choice depends on the severity and frequency of the headaches, the associated symptoms, the presence of other medical illness, and the person's previous responses to medicine. Oral pain medications, NSAIDs, or caffeine-containing medications are useful for persons with mild-to-moderate headaches. When prescription drugs are indicated, your doctor may add butalbital or Midrin®, the adjunctive medications found in the prescription drug. Although these combinations may be more effective than simple analgesics or NSAIDs, one must be aware of the high addiction potential. Because of the risk of dependency, abuse, and daily headache, analgesic overuse must be avoided.

The major side effects of NSAIDs, including aspirin, are stomach bleeding, nausea, vomiting, constipation, ulcers, epigastric pain, and diarrhea. Be sure to tell your doctor if you have a history of hypersensitivity to aspirin or any NSAID, peptic ulcers, bleeding tendency, or severe renal, cardiac, or liver impairment, or if you are being treated with anticoagulants. People with kidney failure should avoid these medications.

If the frequency and severity of your headache attacks warrant it, your doctor may suggest preventive medication. It may surprise you that this may be an antidepressant, such as Elavil®, the most commonly used

> If the frequency and severity of your headache attacks warrant it, your doctor may suggest preventive medication.

preventive for tension-type headache, or Prozac®. These medications have been shown to be very effective against headache, completely separate from their action against depression.

Muscle relaxants may also be prescribed. Botulinum toxin has recently been shown to be a primary treatment for chronic tension-type headache.

Acupuncture*

An analysis of traditional acupuncture, while suggesting that acupuncture had a role in the treatment of headache, found that the evidence was unconvincing. Among recent studies, three showed no benefit and one showed benefit comparable to medication. Some people benefit from acupuncture.

Physical Therapy

Physical therapy consists of heat, cold packs, ultrasound, and electrical stimulation; improvement of posture through stretching, exercise, and traction; and trigger point injections, or occipital nerve blocks. Eating a balanced diet, adequate sleep, and regular exercise and stretching make sense for all of us. Physical therapy may be warranted for people who have tension-type headache associated with muscle spasm or tightness.

---

* The nonmedication therapies discussed in this section are also discussed in Chapter 8.

> Eating a balanced diet, adequate sleep, and
> regular exercise and stretching make sense
> for all of us.

Psychological Factors

Your psychological health may also be addressed, because depression, anxiety, or both may accompany or aggravate tension-type headache. If

> Your psychological health may also be
> addressed, because depression, anxiety, or
> both may accompany or aggravate tension
> headache.

so, these conditions—which are often consequences rather than causes of the headache—need to be appropriately treated. Treatments may include counseling, stress management, relaxation therapy, biofeedback, or medication.

Biofeedback

EMG biofeedback enables people to control muscle tension by providing continuous information about the tension in one or more of the muscles. The feedback can be auditory—for example, clicks that vary in rate, or visual, such as bars that vary in length. Sessions last about one hour. The treatment starts to work when people learn to either increase or decrease their head EMG activity.

Relaxation Training

Progressive relaxation training and autogenic training are both helpful for people with tension-type headaches. Progressive relaxation training helps people recognize tension and relax by sequentially tensing and then releasing (relaxing) various groups of muscles throughout the body. Relaxation training is practiced daily at home and audiotapes are usually provided for assistance. Autogenic training is based on autosuggestion. It seeks to simultaneously regulate mental and body functions by passively concentrating on a positive phrase such as, "My forehead is cool."

Cognitive-Behavioral Therapy

The goal of cognitive therapy is to teach people to identify and challenge dysfunctional thoughts and, subsequently, the underlying maladaptive assumptions and beliefs. Cognitive behavioral interventions, such as stress management programs, may effectively reduce tension-type headaches, but they usually work best in conjunction with biofeedback or relaxation therapies, particularly for people who experience a high level of daily stress. These treatments have been shown to be effective and often improve the results of drug treatment.

CHAPTER 10

Cluster Headaches

T HE WORD *CLUSTER* REFERS to the series of attacks that are characteristic of episodic cluster headache. The cycles of daily, multiple, short-duration headaches that last 1 to 4 months are separated by remissions that last 6 to 24 months.

Only one person in a thousand is unfortunate enough to experience cluster headaches. Of these, three-fourths are men. They are often smokers and are (or have been) heavy drinkers.

> Only one person in a thousand is unfortunate enough to experience cluster headaches. Of these, three-fourths are men. They are often smokers and are (or have been) heavy drinkers.

Cluster headache attacks are one-sided. The pain is located around the eye, temple, or upper jaw and it is excruciating. It is often described as feeling like "a hot poker in the eye." The attacks last from 15 to 90 minutes, occur one to four times daily, and often awaken the person after $1\frac{1}{2}$ to 2 hours of sleep. The attacks often occur at precisely the same time each day. The eye may water and become reddened and the eyelid may droop. Facial or eyelid swelling, nasal stuffiness, and runny nose on the side of the headache may also be present. While migraineurs tend to be quiet and want to lie down in a dark, quiet room, cluster headache pain may be aggravated by lying down. Cluster headache sufferers commonly become agitated. They typically pace the floor, rock back and forth, or even bang their head against a wall during an attack (Figure 10-1).

129

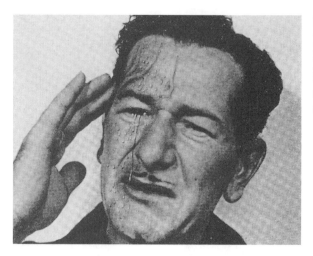

FIGURE 10-1

Patients with cluster headache have been known to injure themselves during an attack.

In summary, cluster headache is one-sided, excruciatingly painful, and accompanied by eye redness, tearing, drooping of the eyelid, and stuffiness of the nostril on the side of the headache; it is more common in men. Most people have episodic cluster headache. The disorder is called *chronic cluster headache* if the attacks continue for one year without remission.

CAUSES OF CLUSTER HEADACHE

The clock-like regularity of cluster attacks, occurring each day at a particular time or at particular seasons, suggests that it is a disorder that involves a part of the brain known as the *hypothalamus*, the brain's clock.

> The clock-like regularity of cluster attacks, occurring each day at a particular time or at particular seasons, suggests that it is a disorder that involves a part of the brain known as the *hypothalamus*, the brain's clock.

Recent neuroimaging studies using positron emission tomography, which measures the activity of the brain, show that the hypothalamus is activated during an attack. The pain is due to activation of the *trigeminal nerve*, which is responsible for sensation on most of the head and around the eye. The runny nose, sweating, and eyelid swelling of a cluster headache are due to activation of a part of the nervous system known as the *parasympathetic system*. Swelling around the carotid artery behind the eye can damage another part of the nervous system called the *sympathetic nervous system*. This can cause some people to have a droopy eyelid and small pupil on the cluster side (Figure 10-2).

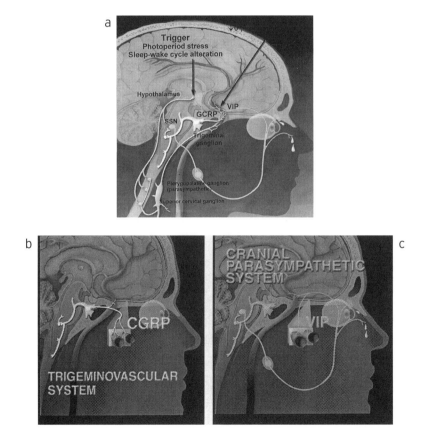

FIGURE 10-2

Brain areas involved in cluster headache. (a) Multiple triggers can start the cluster attack by activating the hypothalamus, the part of the brain responsible for sleep and waking. (b) Activation of the trigeminal nerve releases substances responsible for pain (CGRP). (c) Cranial parasympathetic activation releases a substance responsible for tearing (VIP).

Frank is a 25-year-old smoker who had severe headaches for several days as he drove home after ending his shift at 4:30 p.m. The headaches always occurred over his right eye; they were excruciating and lasted one hour. His right eye would tear and his right nostril was stuffy. When he got home, he could not sit still and he paced rapidly. His wife noted that his eye looked swollen and his whole eye was red during an attack. If she approached her husband, he would get angry and yell at her. By the weekend, Frank was getting two attacks, one in the afternoon and one waking him up two hours after he fell asleep. He also had an attack after consuming alcohol.

Frank went to the emergency room, was seen by two doctors, and saw a chiropractor, who treated him for "migraine." After two months, the headaches went away, but resumed the next year, on precisely the day they had started the year before. After just one headache, he was so terrified that when they occur he goes to the emergency room and refuses to leave until he speaks to "an expert."

This story illustrates the severity and the precise regularity of the attacks that many cluster headache sufferers experience. Note that if this headache had occurred during work hours, Frank would have been unable to work during the attacks and for awhile afterwards, as he recovered from the pain. Because the attacks occurred in the evenings, he had a good attendance record at work, although he was probably fatigued from lack of sleep and coping with his headaches.

Frank's cluster attacks are typical for age of onset, presence of smoking, male gender, number of attacks per day, and agitated behavior (unlike the passive behavior of a migraine sufferer). Frank is "lucky" it only took a year to get an accurate diagnosis, because it often takes several.

TREATMENT OF CLUSTER HEADACHE

Cluster headache is a medical emergency. Because of the incredible pain and the desperate knowledge that the pain will recur again and again, people need rapid and effective treatment. Before effective treatments were available, cluster headache was known as the *suicide headache*. Naturally, the desperation is particularly severe in persons with a chronic cluster headache condition.

Cluster headache is a medical emergency. Because of the incredible pain and the desperate knowledge that the pain will recur again and again, people need rapid and effective treatment.

Maintenance Therapy

Preventive treatment should be started as soon as possible during the cluster period, because it may not be effective until drugs have been used at sufficient doses for one or two weeks (see Table 10-1).

Preventive treatment should be started as soon as possible during the cluster period, because it may not be effective until drugs have been used at sufficient doses for one or two weeks.

TABLE 10-1 Preventive Treatment for Cluster Headache

Short-Term Use Episodic Cluster Headache	Long-Term Use Episodic Cluster Headache Prolonged Chronic Cluster Headache
• Corticosteroids (prednisolone, prednisone, and dexamethasone) • Daily (nocturnal) ergotamine • Greater occipital nerve block	• Verapamil • Lithium • Divalproex sodium • Topiramate • Melatonin*

*Unproven but promising

The drugs that are commonly used for preventive cluster therapy include verapamil (Calan® and Veralen®), lithium carbonate, divalproex (Depakote®), and topiramate (Topamax®). Ergotamine is used for nighttime attacks. Other possibly effective treatments include olanzapine and capsaicin cream—extracted from chili peppers—which is rubbed inside the nose.

A surgical treatment that involves placing an implantable brain stimulator in the hypothalamus has recently been developed to treat chronic cluster sufferers who have severe, one-sided pain. In the past, this surgical procedure generally involved damaging the sensory nerve to the eye. Most recently, an occipital nerve stimulator has been found to be effective. Surgical procedures are reserved for people for whom all preventive therapy has failed.

Transitional Treatment

Transitional treatment can be used to bridge the gap before preventive drugs take effect. Commonly used agents include corticosteroids (prednisone) and dihydroergotamine. Corticosteroids (Prednisone® and Medrol®) provide rapid relief, but while they are relatively safe in the short term, their long-term use may result in severe adverse side-effects, such as bone loss, muscle weakness, and increased abdominal fat. Repetitive intravenous dihydroergotamine can be used to break an attack of intractable cluster headache. Occipital nerve block utilizing a local analgesic and a corticosteroid on the side of the headache is effective in about two-thirds of those with cluster. A nerve block of a cluster of cells accessible through the nose (*pterygopalatine ganglia*) is available in some centers.

Acute Therapy

Cluster headache may occur despite appropriate transitional or maintenance therapy. Acute therapies, used to shorten or abort the cluster attack, should be administered when symptoms begin (see Table 10-2). They may resolve an individual cluster attack, but will not prevent further attacks. Giving 100 percent oxygen for 10 minutes via a mask is a safe and effective method of aborting a cluster headache attack. However, oxygen treatment often merely postpones the attack.

Subcutaneous sumatriptan (Imitrex®) and intramuscular or intravenous dihydroergotamine are very effective in aborting cluster headache

> Giving 100 percent oxygen for 10 minutes via a mask is a safe and effective method of aborting a cluster headache attack.

attacks, but use of these drugs should be limited to twice a day. Dihydroergotamine is the one medication that may prevent further attacks. By and large, pain medicines, including opioids, are relatively ineffective for cluster headache.

TABLE 10-2 Abortive Treatment for Cluster Headache

Treatment	Efficacy	Tolerability	Clinical Use
100 percent oxygen (7-12 L/min) for 15 to 20 min	Aborts headache in 70 percent in less than 15 minutes	Very well-tolerated	First line choice; inconvenient
Sumatriptan 20 mg intranasally	Effective	Triptan adverse events;	First line choice
Sumatriptan 6 mg subcutaneously	Highly effective	contraindicated in cardiovascular disease	First line choice
Dihydroergotamine 1.0 mg or intravenously	Highly effective intramuscularly	Contraindicated in cardiovascular disease	First line choice
Lidocaine intranasally (4 to 6 percent)	Questionable	Fair to good	Limited

CHAPTER 11

Unusual Headaches

PAROXYSMAL HEMICRANIA

PAROXYSMAL HEMICRANIA IS A VERY RARE, cluster-like headache that predominantly affects women. Similar to cluster headaches, the attacks occur on one side only, are centered in the area around the eye, and are excruci-

> *Paroxysmal hemicrania* is a very rare, cluster-like headache that predominantly affects women.

atingly painful. They are accompanied by prominent tearing, drooping of the eyelid, and facial swelling on the side of the headache. The main differences between paroxysmal hemicrania and cluster headache are that the attacks are much briefer (15 minutes as opposed to one hour) and more frequent (usually more than six times a day). This type of attack is similar to cluster headache and can be both acute and chronic. Unlike cluster headache, paroxysmal hemicrania is well-controlled by indomethacin.

CHRONIC DAILY HEADACHE

There are four types of chronic daily headache: chronic tension-type headache, chronic migraine, new daily persistent headache, and *hemicrania continua*. All occur more than 15 days a month and last more than four hours a day. Since chronic tension-type headache and chronic migraine were discussed in previous chapters, they will not be discussed here.

HEMICRANIA CONTINUA

Hemicrania continua is the least common of these four headache types. It is a continuous, one-sided headache of moderate severity, with periods of worsening of symptoms when the pain becomes severe. It may be accompanied by nausea, sensitivity to light and sound, tearing, redness of the eye, and droopy eyelid. Eye discomfort has been described, and some people report a feeling of sand in the eye.

Hemicrania continua exists in both continuous and remitting (comes and goes) forms. The continuous variety can be continuous from the start or evolve from the remitting variety. The remitting bouts last from 1 to 6 months, separated by pain-free periods of 2 weeks to 6 months. This disorder almost always responds to indomethacin.

The cause of hemicrania continua is unknown. It is one of several indomethacin-responsive headaches that have a special sensitivity to this medication. A diagnosis of hemicrania continua may not be certain until indomethacin is tried, because this disorder may have features of both migraine and cluster headaches.

> A diagnosis of hemicrania continua may not be certain until indomethacin is tried, because this disorder may have features of both migraine and cluster headaches.

Some people cannot tolerate indomethacin because of stomach irritation. There is also a higher risk of kidney damage with this medicine than with other medicines in the same class (nonsteroidal anti-inflammatory drugs [NSAIDs]). Occasionally, indomethacin makes people feel tired or generally ill. For these reasons, physicians sometimes have to settle for another, often less effective NSAID that has fewer side effects and potential risks. Some people have done quite well on the newest subclass of NSAIDs (COX2 inhibitors), particularly rofecoxib (Vioxx®) and celecoxib (Celebrex®).

NEW DAILY PERSISTENT HEADACHE

New daily persistent headache is a more recently defined subtype of chronic daily headache. New daily persistent headache starts suddenly and continues with constant, unremitting pain. It is usually continuous, although some people have headache-free time lasting hours or days. People with this condition do not have a history of worsening tension-type headache or migraine.

The cause of new daily persistent headache is unknown. It generally starts on a particular day, although it may develop over three days. Frequently, no inciting event can be identified. In one-third of the people affected, it begins around the time of a flu-like illness. A virus called *Epstein-Barr*, which is responsible for mononucleosis, may be one cause. It starts around the time of surgery to some part of the body other than the head in 1 of 8 individuals. It also starts at the time of a stressful event in 1 out of 8. It most commonly starts in the 20s in women and in the 40s in men; most sufferers are women. MRI of the brain is almost always normal.

Many people with new daily persistent headache experience symptoms common to migraine: nausea, light and sound sensitivity, and pul-

> Many people with new daily persistent headache experience symptoms common to migraine: nausea, light and sound sensitivity, and pulsating head pain.

sating head pain. A few even experience aura-like symptoms, including zigzag lines and numbness. Aggravating factors are similar to migraine and include stress, exertion, weather changes, bright lights, and menstruation.

There is no specific treatment for new daily persistent headache. It is treated as if it were the headache that it most resembles—if it has the symptoms of chronic migraine, doctors treat it as a migraine, and if it has the features of tension-type headache, doctors treat it as a tension-type headache. In general, new daily persistent headache is somewhat more difficult to treat than transformed migraine or chronic tension-type headache.

> *Amy, a 25-year-old woman, had a few tension-type headaches until one morning two years ago, when she awoke with what she thought was another tension-type headache. By afternoon, the headache was severe, and by the next day, she had a severe bilateral headache with light and sound sensitivity. She was unable to work for three days and then the headache moderated to the point where she had a daily headache that was 5/10 in intensity, involving the whole head, with severe exacerbations including nausea and light sensitivity twice a week. She now misses work twice a month and rarely participates in optional activities. She has had an MRI, a spinal tap, and many blood tests, including a Lyme test, all of which were normal. She has seen several specialists.*

This is a typical story describing new daily persistent headache. Although the disorder is poorly understood, there is little chance that further testing will show a cause. Because the headache has features of migraine as well as of tension-type headache, it should be treated in the same way as chronic migraine, although its prognosis is somewhat worse than that of chronic migraine. Medication overuse must be avoided.

"ICE PICK" HEADACHE

Some people get brief, sudden, severe jabs of pain that resolve completely in a few seconds. The onset of this type of pain is almost instantaneous, but it resolves in as little as one second or it may linger for as long as 30 seconds. This kind of pain usually occurs as part of another type of headache disorder, such as migraine or cluster headache. Occasionally, it occurs by itself when there is no other headache. It usually is quite infrequent, occurring at most a few times a day, but in rare instances, it occurs frequently throughout the day and thus requires treatment.

Because the pain is so peculiar and severe, people are often sure that some physical change or problem must be causing it. In fact, it is rare for any cause, such as a tumor, to be found. Some headache experts believe that if this type of headache is present, it virtually assures that there is no need to look for a cause.

The pain is much too brief to be treated when it occurs. It can usually be prevented by taking indomethacin, although it comes back as soon as the medicine is stopped. Usually only reassurance is needed; it is almost never a long-lasting or chronic problem.

SEXUAL ACTIVITY HEADACHE

Headache that occurs during sexual intercourse or masturbation is called *coital headache*. The most common type is an explosively sudden and severe headache occurring at or around the time of orgasm. This type of headache can be very debilitating and last for hours. Because the nature of the pain is very similar to the headache that occurs as the result of a ruptured *brain aneurysm*, and because intercourse is a well-recognized trigger for rupture of a brain aneurysm, the first time it occurs, a person should be very carefully evaluated to rule out a bleeding aneurysm. This usually involves a CT scan and a spinal tap, which should be done as soon as possible after the headache. If the spinal tap is not done within a few days, a more invasive test that involves inserting a catheter into the blood vessels that go to the brain may be necessary. Most coital headaches are benign and can be treated once a dangerous aneurysm is ruled out.

The pain of the benign, explosive form of coital headache generally resolves within hours. It may or may not recur and sometimes occurs with each sexual activity. It can be prevented by taking indomethacin

> The pain of the benign, explosive form of coital headache generally resolves within hours.

prior to intercourse. Migraine preventive drugs are sometimes effective and *must* be taken daily.

There are two other types of coital headache. One builds up slowly, has the symptoms of an exercise-induced migraine, and is treated as migraine. Another, extremely rare type behaves similar to a positional headache. It is due to leakage of cerebrospinal fluid from a tear in the lining of the spinal canal, and most people improve spontaneously. Treatment involves finding the location of the leak and surgically fixing it.

CHAPTER 12

Nonheadache Illnesses that Frequently Accompany Headache

Psychological Disturbances

THE RELATIONSHIP BETWEEN psychological disorders and headache is complex, and there is little evidence that such a relationship exists, except for migraine.

Depression, anxiety, and migraine have an odd relationship. While migraine is by no means an indication of depression or anxiety—most migraineurs usually do not suffer from either symptom—persons who have migraine are three times as likely to have depression as those who do not have migraine. Similarly, anxiety (including panic) is much more common in migraine sufferers than in nonmigraineurs.

It works the other way as well. Depressed people without migraine are more likely to develop migraine in the future than are people who are not depressed. This relationship has been called *bidirectional*. There may be an underlying, perhaps genetic, predisposition to the development of migraine and depression in some people. The authors believe that if someone has migraine and severe depression or anxiety, treating the headache alone will not be effective in relieving the pain until the psychological problems are addressed.

FIBROMYALGIA

People with *fibromyalgia* have chronic, fluctuating, muscular-type pain in various parts of their bodies, such as the neck and back. They also have tender muscles on examination. Migraine, chronic migraine, and

> People with *fibromyalgia* have chronic, fluctuating, muscular-type pain in various parts of their bodies, such as the neck and back.

chronic tension-type headache are common in people who have fibromyalgia. This may indicate that these disorders share a common hyperexcitability of the pain system.

IRRITABLE BOWEL SYNDROME

Irritable bowel syndrome is another *benign*, painful condition that, similar to fibromyalgia, is common in people who have migraine (and vice versa). These individuals complain of recurrent abdominal pain and often alternating constipation and diarrhea. Testing fails to reveal a cause of the pain.

RESTLESS LEGS SYNDROME

Restless legs syndrome is a condition that causes insomnia due to discomfort in the legs (and occasionally the arms) in the evening and when attempting to sleep. These feelings are accompanied by an irresistible urge to move the limbs. At its worst, it makes it impossible to stay in bed

> *Restless legs syndrome* is a condition that causes insomnia due to discomfort in the legs (and occasionally the arms) in the evening and when attempting to sleep.

for very long before needing to get up and pace. These feelings in the legs and the need to move them make it extremely difficult to fall asleep. People with this condition often need to be completely exhausted before they can fall asleep—before the need to move the legs and the uncomfortable feeling make this impossible.

Restless legs syndrome, experienced before falling asleep, is usually accompanied by periodic leg movements during sleep. These sometimes very subtle movements in the legs are enough to disturb sleep so that the deeper stages of sleep are never reached. Thus even an apparently normal amount of sleep is not restful.

Restless legs syndrome is common in people with migraine and fibromyalgia. This condition can be exacerbated by the antidepressants and antinauseants that are used to treat migraine. The syndrome is often very effectively treated by any one of a variety of medicines taken in the evening or at bedtime. Taking care of restless legs syndrome may be critical if sleep deprivation is exacerbating a headache problem.

RAYNAUD'S PHENOMENON

The hands of a person with Raynaud's phenomenon become white, then pink and purple, and very painful when exposed to cold. Raynaud's and migraine often co-exist. Certain headache medications may exacerbate Raynaud's phenomenon.

SECTION IV

Secondary Headache

CHAPTER 13

Sinus Headache and Nasal Disease

"I don't get migraines; I get sinus headaches."

"Oh, I have such a sinus headache! It must be the weather change."

"I get sinusitis every year at this time."

HOW MANY TIMES have you heard—or said—something similar to the above? Many people are absolutely convinced that their headaches are the result of *sinusitis*. "The pain is right here," they say, pressing their fingers just below the inner corners of their eyes. "I can feel the swelling, and when I press here, it feels better. That's sinusitis, right?"

Acute sinusitis is an infection of one or more of the cranial sinuses (air-filled spaces in the skull). Many migraine and tension-type headaches masquerade as sinusitis, and people are often doggedly con-

> Many migraine and tension-type headaches masquerade as sinusitis.

vinced that they suffer from sinusitis because they believe that pain over the sinuses must be related to the sinuses. Actually, frontal head pain is usually caused by migraine or tension-type headache. Nasal stuffiness is common in migraine, and this bolsters the belief that sinusitis is the culprit (Figure 13-1).

Acute sinusitis affects more than 31 million people in the United States, and the problem is increasing, according to data from the National Ambulatory Medical Care Survey.

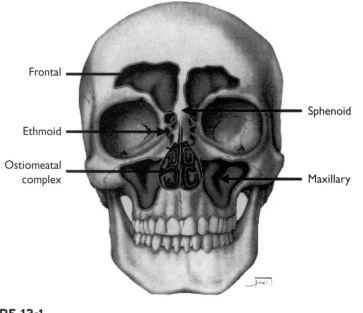

FIGURE 13-1

The paranasal sinuses.

The most common sites of sinus infection in children are the *maxillary sinuses*, located under the cheeks, and the *ethmoid* sinuses, located behind the nose. These sinuses are present at birth. The *sphenoid sinus*, located deep in the head, does not develop until after the age of two years, and it does not start to contain air until the child is approximately eight years of age. The frontal sinuses, located above the eyes, develop at about six years of age. These frontal and sphenoid sinuses are frequent sites of infection among teenagers, when the accessory sinuses of the nose become inflamed.

CAUSE OF SINUSITIS

Obstruction of the entrance to the sinuses is the major cause of sinusitis. The sinuses are air-filled cavities that connect with the nasal passages, which warm and humidify the air as we breathe. These cavities are lined with cells that contain hair-like projections, which are in turn covered by a thin layer of mucus. The hair-like structures move in a way that creates a flow of mucus out of the sinuses into the nasal cavity. When this flow is stopped, sinusitis—and that all-too-familiar "stuffed up" feeling—is often the result.

DIAGNOSTIC TESTING

Computed Tomography

Computed tomography (CT) is the best study to evaluate the sinuses. A CT scan may show thickening of the surface of the sinuses, scarring, clouding, or air-fluid levels (as in a glass of water). Reversible sinus abnormalities are often seen on CT in people suffering from the common cold. This suggests that CT may not be able to diagnose bacterial infections, but only the presence of inflammation, which could be due to a virus or bacteria (Figure 13-2).

Nasal Endoscopy

The doctor can use a flexible fiberoptic instrument to look inside the nose and visualize the nasal passages and sinus drainage areas to easily

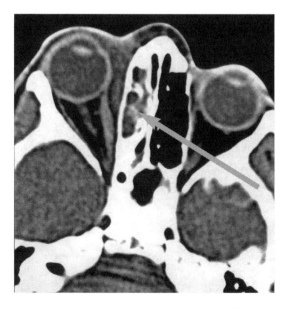

FIGURE 13-2

CT scan of a person with sinusitis shows the presence of inflammation. Dark black areas are normal sinuses, filled with air; shades of white and gray (arrow) indicate the presence of inflammatory tissue in the sinuses, where none should be.

determine whether infection *is* present. If infection is present, pus will be seen coming from the openings of the sinuses. Mucosal sinus thickening is frequently present in individuals who do not have any symptoms due to sinus changes. In these cases, the doctor should visualize the nasal structures before making a diagnosis of sinusitis.

RHINOSINUSITIS

In 1996, the American Academy of Head and Neck Surgery chose the word *rhinosinusitis* over *sinusitis* because rhinitis, an inflammation of the nasal structures, typically precedes sinusitis. It is rare to have infectious sinusitis without rhinitis. This makes sense because the tissues of the nose and sinuses are connected, and symptoms of nasal obstruction and discharge are a prominent part of sinusitis. The diagnosis of rhinosinusitis is usually based on symptoms indicating maxillary or frontal sinus involvement. Rhinosinusitis is divided into four categories (see Table 13-1).

Tenderness and pain of the face, nasal congestion, and nasal discharge in the form of pus are commonly seen in acute sinus infection. Other signs and symptoms include an inability to smell, pain upon chewing, and *halitosis* (bad breath). Headache, facial pain, and fever may not be present. Upper jaw toothache, poor response to decongestants, purulent discharge (pus), and colored nasal discharge can all indicate sinusitis.

The pain of sinusitis results from swollen and inflamed nasal structures. Sinus headache usually has a deep, dull, aching quality combined with a heaviness and fullness. Nausea and vomiting are rare. Migraine

TABLE 13-1 Categories of Rhinosinusitis

Acute rhinosinusitis is sudden in onset, lasts from one day to four weeks, and symptoms resolve completely.

Subacute rhinosinusitis lasts from 4 to 12 weeks.

Recurrent acute rhinosinusitis requires four or more episodes of acute rhinosinusitis, lasting at least 7 days each, in any one-year period.

Chronic rhinosinusitis means the signs or symptoms persist for 12 weeks or longer and may be punctuated by acute infectious episodes. Most experts do not believe this exists.

> Sinus headache usually has a deep, dull, aching quality combined with a heaviness and fullness.

and tension-type headaches are often confused with true sinus headaches because of similarity in location. Most headache doctors and many ear, nose, and throat doctors believe that chronic rhinosinusitis is rarely a cause of headache.

DEVIATED SEPTUM HEADACHE

Rarely, a deviated septum may cause a one-sided headache on the side toward which septum deviates. If the septal deviation is causing the headache, placing a small piece of paper soaked in an anesthetic (lidocaine or Novocaine®) will relieve the headache. The treatment is surgical straightening of the deviated sinus.

SINUS HEADACHE TREATMENT

The management goals for the treatment of sinusitis are listed in Table 13-2. Uncomplicated sinusitis, other than sphenoid sinusitis, is treated with antibiotics for 10 to 14 days. Sphenoid sinusitis can be much more dangerous and may need more aggressive, prolonged treatment.

Inhalation of steam and saline prevent crusting of secretions and help clear mucus from the nose. Decongestants relieve symptoms by shrinking inflamed and swollen nasal tissues. They should only be used for 3 to 4 days in order to prevent decongestant rebound (swelling when

---

TABLE 13-2 Treatment Goals for Sinusitis

• Treat bacterial infection

• Reduce *ostial* swelling

• Drain sinuses

• Maintain *sinus ostia patency*

decongestant use is delayed or stopped). Decongestants should be taken by mouth if treatment for more than three days is necessary. These agents reduce nasal blood flow without the risk of rebound vasodilation.

Antihistamines are not effective in the management of acute rhinitis. Anti-inflammatory topical corticosteroids may help maintain open passages from the sinuses into the nasal passageways.

CONFUSING MIGRAINE WITH SINUS HEADACHE

Most migraineurs experience some kind of sinus pressure during a migraine attack. Many believe, therefore, that they have sinus headache. Others believe they must be having sinus headache because weather changes trigger their attacks. In fact, weather changes trigger

> Most migraineurs experience some kind of sinus pressure during a migraine attack. Many believe, therefore, that they have sinus headache.

migraine, *not* sinus headache. In general, finding migraines among persons who think they have sinus headache is easy and it turns out to be almost everyone. Nausea, light and sound sensitivity, and even neck pain points to migraine and away from a process within the nose or sinuses. The illusion exists because there is tissue swelling within the nose as part of migraine headache, and even more so in cluster headache. Many of the drugs that treat sinus headache actually help migraines a little and also cause rebound headache. Unfortunately, the myth of sinus headache has prevented many people from being appropriately diagnosed and treated.

CHAPTER 14

Disorders
of the Neck

"It doesn't happen every time, but that's the only time it does happen."

"What are you talking about, Alice?"

"My headaches! It's so weird! They only happen when I tilt my head like this...."

"Well, don't do it, for God's sake! You'll get a headache!"

"No, no! That's what I was trying to say. It doesn't happen every time I tilt my head. I'd be going crazy! But that's the only time I do get a headache!"

"You're strange, Alice."

Lewis Carroll, Alice in Wonderland

ACTUALLY, THE FICTIONAL ALICE in the above conversation is not so strange at all. She probably suffers from what is called *cervicogenic headache*. As the name implies, this is a headache that is generated in the neck. Moving or holding the neck in certain positions is the only thing (other than the

> Moving or holding the neck in certain positions is the only thing (other than the occasional sneeze or cough) that will bring on a cervicogenic headache.

occasional sneeze or cough) that will bring on a cervicogenic headache. The pain starts in the back of the head and may spread forward. It never switches sides. Cervicogenic headache may be due to dystonia or it may be a disorder unto itself. Most people with headache and pain in the neck have referred pain due to migraine or tension-type headache. Over half of migraineurs have neck pain during an attack. However, headache can also be caused by problems in the neck (Figure 14-1).

Many parts of the neck are sensitive to pain: the joints between the vertebrae, the periosteum (bone lining), ligaments of the cervical spine, the neck muscles, the cervical nerves, and the vertebral arteries and veins of the cervical spine. Pain can arise from all of these. Neck discomfort, stiffness, or pain may extend into the shoulders, the upper arms, and into the forearms and fingers. It may also be referred to various regions of the head, even the eyes. Headache may be present on awakening or may begin after coming home from work, and may last several hours. Later, the pain can become continuous, but even then it manifests diurnal variations in intensity. The pain may start in the neck or the *occiput* (the back of the head) and sweep forward. Some people have pain in the temples; others have neck pain referred to the forehead or one entire half of the head; and some have bilateral pain. Crunching sounds in the neck (*crepitus*) may be heard.

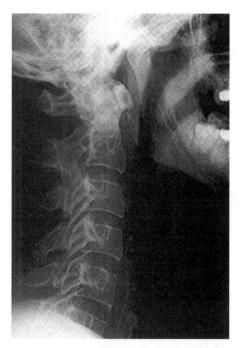

FIGURE 14-1

Cervical spine X-ray showing straightening of the neck due to muscle spasm. Muscle spasms can trigger head pain.

Headache referred from the neck has many causes. People with this type of headache may be born with joint hypermobility or congenital neck joint fusion. Trauma, particularly whiplash injury in car accidents, and even neck hyperextension after *tracheal* tube placement during operations, can occasionally bring on this type of headache. Maintaining one neck position for a long period of time is common in various occupations, especially musicians, typists, video display unit workers, and word processor operators, making these professions vulnerable to this type of headache. However, the most common problem that physicians see arises from aging joints in the neck. Most of us experience crunching sounds when we move our necks, or limitation of neck mobility as we get older.

Developmental *anomalies* (abnormalities you were born with) of the junction between the head and upper cervical spine frequently cause headaches. *Occipital* or *suboccipital* pain occurs in about a quarter of people with *basilar invagination* (abnormal bones of the head), *Arnold-Chiari malformation*, where the back of the brain extends downward into the spinal canal, and other disorders. There is nothing specific about these headaches, but they often have features, such as posterior location, that are triggered by flexing of the neck or coughing and straining. There is sometimes a pronounced postural component that worsens with standing and is relieved by lying down. People with this condition may have vertigo, facial numbness, weakness of arms or legs, or ataxia (an inability to coordinate muscle activity during involuntary movement), as well as neurologic findings that the doctor would look for. Surgery rarely helps people with these abnormalities unless they have cough headache or neurologic symptoms.

Problems can develop in the *craniovertebral* junction and upper cervical spine, such as tumors, *osteomyelitis* (bone infection), and *multiple myeloma* (a blood cancer). They produce headache by eroding the pain-sensitive structures or putting traction on upper cervical nerve roots. Blows to the head or even forceful sneezing may produce problems in the cervical vertebrae, which can in turn cause persistent occipital headache. Rheumatoid arthritis of the upper cervical spine produces headaches because of inflammation of the synovial joints and stretching

> Rheumatoid arthritis of the upper cervical spine produces headaches because of inflammation of the synovial joints and stretching of the neck ligaments and nerves.

of the neck ligaments and nerves. These disorders produce occipital headaches that are worsened or triggered by neck movements or straining, but the postural element of the headache is not so evident.

Arthritis of the bones of the neck (*cervical spondylosis*) is not completely accepted as a cause of headache. First, this is very common over the age of 40 years. Second, it mainly involves the lower neck and does not usually cause head pain. However, the restriction of movement in these lower cervical regions possibly leads to excessive "play" in the upper neck, and this could cause headache. Unconsciously, the body tries to maintain its normal movement patterns. In order to balance the restricted movement of the lower neck, movement of the upper portion may increase. This increased movement may produce headache, typically in the back of the head, and often on one side.

Trauma, including whiplash injuries to the neck, can cause headache. Many people with an extension-flexion injury of the neck have self-limited neck, occipital, and occasionally frontal pain that clears

> Trauma, including whiplash injuries to the neck, can cause headache.

within days or a few weeks. This pain results from injury to the upper cervical ligaments and muscles. Headaches that last months or years are more difficult to explain. Shearing injuries of the long axons in the brainstem and upper cord may disrupt central pain and other resultant mechanisms, allowing the emergence of headache. This type of mechanism could account for the typical migraine that follows some whiplash injuries, which responds well to prophylactic antimigraine medication.

As discussed in Chapter 7 and also above, *dystonia* is a muscle spasm that bends and twists the neck. It is not a disease in itself, but is a syndrome diagnosis, similar to a headache. The common central symptom of focal dystonia is the abnormal movements or defective position of the affected parts of the body. Focal dystonia occurring in the head and neck region is called *craniocervical dystonia* (CCD) (Figure 14-2). This condition is often encountered in middle-aged adults. The underlying muscular hyperactivity may rise to a slow, smooth movement or a fixed defective position; it may cause jerky, repetitive movement or it may be rhythmic, similar to a tremor. Pain is common in dystonia of the neck. It is either due to continuous contraction of muscles or a result of nerve irritation caused by the muscular hyperactivity.

Cervical spine disorders are believed to be a fairly common cause of headache, because often pain is located in the neck and back of the head. Confusing the matter is the fact that neck pain is present in most migraine and many tension-type headaches. A diagnosis of headache caused by a neck disorder requires the satisfaction of the following specific criteria:

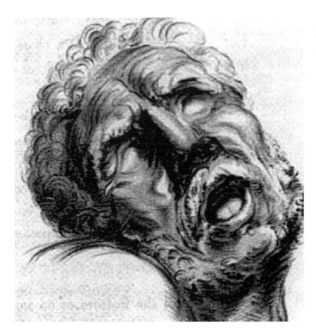

FIGURE 14-2

Dystonia can cause headache.

- The headache must occur in the neck and back of the head region, but radiation to other parts of the head or neck is possible.
- The headache may occur on either one or both sides.
- It must be possible to provoke the pain by means of particular neck movements or particular positions.
- The doctor's examination should reveal evidence of restricted movement, changes in structure, contour or tone of cervical muscles, or increased sensitivity to pain on palpation.
- An X-ray of the cervical spine often reveals a straightened neck with loss of normal curvature due to muscle spasm, as well as spondylosis (arthritis).

Sometimes something serious may be going on in the neck that may also cause headache. If you find yourself tilting your head to one side, or the rotation of your head on your neck is limited—and especially if it is painful—or your ability to move your upper neck front and back is decreased, your doctor may order a computed tomography scan (CT) or magnetic resonance imaging (MRI). Plain X-rays of the skull base rarely are adequate.

Therapy always starts with a thorough investigation to identify a cause. The usual treatments for cervicogenic headache are physical in nature. Muscle tenderness may be eased or increased by pressing on the

> The usual treatments for cervicogenic headache are physical in nature.

tender muscle with your fingers. A hot shower gives temporary relief. Mobilization, manipulation, massage, deep heat, and other physical methods often give comfort. Some may find a cervical collar helpful. At first, it may have to be worn both day and night. However, too much use can lead to stiffness, weak muscles, and pain. A firm foam pad under the pillow or a shaped foam pillow is often used (*cervical pillow*). The usual recommended pharmaceutical treatment is nonsteroidal anti-inflammatory drugs (NSAIDs). Some people need antidepressants, sedatives, or muscle relaxants. Occasionally, your doctor may use a local anesthetic block to relieve the pain (trigger point injections or nerve blocks of the C2 root or greater occipital nerve). Occipital nerve blocks are also used to treat cluster headache and some cases of migraine. Botulinum toxin (Botox®) is used to treat some kinds of cervicogenic headache.

A 56-year-old man who sat in front of a computer for at least half of his working day complained of right-sided headache for several years. He awakened most days with pain, but it usually dissipated after he showered, shaved, and had breakfast, only to recur when he sat and watched television in the evening. The headache sometimes persisted for the whole day and, on occasion, it awakened him in the early morning hours.

The pain started in his neck and spread over his ear to his forehead. Stretching his neck or massaging it helped, but his neck movements were limited. When the pain was moderate, two pain-relieving tablets reduced or abolished the symptoms in about 30 minutes.

He had no past neck or whiplash injury, but he had been a boxer in college.

Examination showed restricted neck movements in rotation and lateral bending. The neck muscles were tender bilaterally, more on the right than the left, and the right trapezius muscle was tender on palpation.

X-rays of the neck showed minor spondylosis *(joint stiffening or fixation) and loss of the normal* lordosis *(curvature of the spinal column).*

He was treated with moist heat followed by stretching, and had an excellent result.

CHAPTER 15

Post-Traumatic
Headache

Heather Kelly was bright, beautiful, and only 22 years old. The world was an exciting place. She was just out of college, newly married, and working at a job in her chosen career. One day, she was on her way back to the office after lunch, invigorated by the very tempo of working in the center of a major city, when from far above a huge window pane fell from a skyscraper, hitting her on the head, rendering her unconscious and knocking her to the ground.

She seemed to be one giant ache when she woke up. Cuts and bruises covered her body; her face was stitched together; and much of her beautiful blonde hair had been shaved away. In less than a heartbeat, her life had changed radically.

Strong and determined, Heather survived, and even triumphed. Her hair grew back. Plastic surgeons repaired her face. Her scars healed. Only one thing remained to remind her of her ordeal, as if she could forget! She was troubled by excruciating headaches. She would wake during the night, feeling as if an iron band was being tightened around her head. Nothing she took or did lessened her pain.

POST-TRAUMATIC HEADACHE, defined as headache following head trauma, is one of the most controversial types of headaches. Some experts believe that it has been fabricated by lawyers and greed. Others consider it a biological disorder resulting from permanent brain or nerve

> Post-traumatic headache, defined as headache following head trauma, is one of the most controversial types of headaches.

injury. No one can deny that it generates a huge amount of medical, legal, and insurance company activity.

Post-traumatic headache is similar to other headache disorders in that it has both acute and chronic forms. No one questions the existence of acute post-traumatic headache, a new headache (as opposed to worsening of a previous headache problem) that begins within one week of a blow or jarring movement of the head. It may be accompanied by nausea, light and sound sensitivity, and other features of migraine. Concentration and memory problems are common, and people with post-traumatic headache have trouble managing several tasks simultaneously. Vertigo may occur. Sleep disturbances and acquired alcohol intolerance are also common.

While everyone agrees that acute post-traumatic headache is a legitimate biological disorder, chronic post-traumatic headache with symptoms that last many months or become permanent is very controversial. Studies in the United States and Europe suggest that headache is permanent in 20 percent of persons who see a doctor for acute post-traumatic headache. Post-traumatic headache also occurs in Japan and India. However, studies in Lithuania—where there is no compensation for disability after car accidents—do not find the same high incidence of daily headache occurring years after the injury.

It has been suggested that the belief that long-term headache can result after injury actually causes chronic post-traumatic symptoms. The authors disagree that the expectation of symptoms is a major cause of chronic post-traumatic headache. Chronic post-traumatic headache is seen in North America, most of Europe, India, Japan, and many other countries with diverse cultures and legal systems. However, the cause of the post-traumatic headache is undermined by unethical lawyers and a legal system that encourages people who have been in accidents to embellish or manufacture symptoms, and by doctors who order tests and treatments in order to increase bills, thus increasing damage awards.

To qualify as a chronic post-traumatic headache, pain must persist for more than three months. Sleep and mood disturbances are common. Balance, concentration, and memory problems may persist. Resolution of a legal case (if one exists) does not cure the symptoms.

To qualify as a chronic post-traumatic headache, pain must persist for more than three months.

The features of acute and chronic post-traumatic headache usually resemble a "naturally occurring" headache disorder, such as chronic tension-type headache, chronic or transformed migraine, and rarely, cluster headache. Cognitive problems may be subtle, yet profound. Post-traumatic headache sufferers often feel their memory, concentration, and attention spans are very poor. Yet, despite severe difficulties in real life situations, formal testing is usually normal unless very sophisticated tests are performed. The life of the chronic post-traumatic headache sufferer becomes truly miserable because of daily headaches, cognitive problems, legal difficulties, and disbelief by a large portion of society that chronic post-traumatic headache even exists as a legitimate problem.

When a head injury occurs, most of the linear (forward and backward) motion of the body is converted into rotational (circular) movement of the brain, because the neck hinges the head relative to the body and because the brain is more fixed to the skull at its base than on its outside. The nerve axons, which are long, thin, thread-like processes, are stretched, causing immediate injury that produces an alteration in or loss of consciousness (Figure 15-1). The axons are actually cut in more

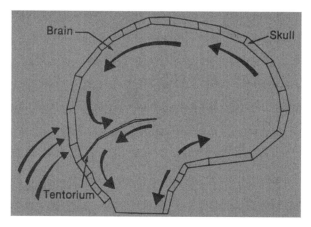

FIGURE 15-1

Movement of the brain in the skull after head injury.

severe cases; in less severe cases, they remain unbroken but do not function normally for a long period of time. Even minor concussions without loss of consciousness can have a long-lasting effect on brain func-

> Even minor concussions without loss of
> consciousness can have a long-lasting effect
> on brain function.

tion. Football players with this kind of concussion do worse academical-
ly than those who have never suffered a concussion. In some people, a
mild acute concussion triggers an immediate visual migraine aura.

The acute post-traumatic headache may start immediately after
injury or within a few days. This is probably due to the stretching of
axons and the subsequent release of brain chemicals into the spaces that
surround the nerves, thereby altering their function. What is less clear is
why the headache and nonheadache symptoms resolve in most people,
but are permanent in some. The severe psychological stress to which
head trauma victims are subjected by society may play a part, but biological factors are almost certainly important as well.

There is no specific treatment for post-traumatic headache. It is
treated according to its symptoms—that is, if the headache behaves in a

> There is no specific treatment for post-
> traumatic headache.

manner similar to chronic migraine, it is treated in the same manner as
a migraine headache. The same applies to post-traumatic headaches that
resemble tension-type or cluster headaches. A neck injury should be
addressed with physical therapy and home exercises. Some individuals,
especially those whose neck has been injured with a whiplash injury
and who have one-sided neck pain radiating to the back of the head,
may have injury to a joint in the neck that is called a *facet*. Anesthetizing
the injured joint temporarily relieves the pain. Once the correct joint is

identified, a procedure called *radiofrequency rhizotomy* can be performed that deadens the nerves to the appropriate joint for about a year, providing excellent relief.

Post-traumatic vertigo is often difficult to treat. Sleep problems may be partially helped with treatment. However, there is a risk in using habit-forming medications. Concentration and memory problems may be addressed by learning strategies that compensate for the problems. Depression must be treated aggressively if it occurs.

CHAPTER 16

Atypical Facial Pain and Trigeminal Neuralgia

M. Alan Stiles, D.M.D.

PEOPLE WHO COMPLAIN OF FACIAL or head pain that does not fit perfectly into other diagnostic categories are often told they have TMJ or
TMD (*temporomandibular joint disorders*). These people have usually seen
multiple caregivers, including their primary care physician, a dentist, an
oral surgeon, a neurologist, a chiropractor, an acupuncturist, or even an
ear, nose, and throat specialist. Each evaluation generates a new opinion and new treatment options and therapies. Quite often, the person
has undergone multiple treatments, yet continues to suffer with the
original complaint. TMJ or TMD becomes the diagnosis for these people,
even though their pain may originate elsewhere (Figure 16-1).

*Mrs. Evans was sitting at her desk when suddenly she felt a jolt of pain in her
lower left jaw. The pain stopped her in her tracks and then was gone as quickly as it had appeared. The pain occurred near a tooth on which she had had a
crown placed in the past few months. Frightened that the pain would return, she
made an appointment with her dentist, who tested the tooth by tapping on it
with a dental instrument; the pain returned a few minutes later. The dentist concluded that the pain must be coming from the tooth, and he performed a root
canal procedure, which he believed would fix the problem.*

*Following the root canal, the pain disappeared for 2 or 3 weeks, but then
returned, just as it was in the beginning. This time the pain occurred 1 to 2 times
a day. She returned to her dentist, who referred her to an endodontist, in case*

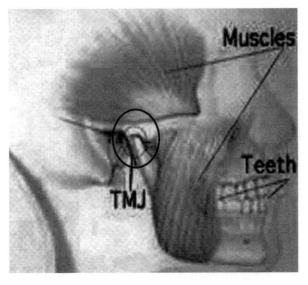

FIGURE 16-1

The temporomadibular joint.

an extra canal needed to be treated. The endodontist repeated the root canal. Mrs. Evans was again pain-free for a few weeks, after which time her pain returned. The endodontist then referred her to an ear, nose, and throat specialist, who concluded it must be TMJ because no abnormality was found on examination. The endodontist then referred Mrs. Evans to an oral surgeon.

Upon examination, the oral surgeon decided that her temporomandibular joints were working normally and he sent her to a neurologist with a diagnosis of possible neuralgia. The neurologist examined Mrs. Evans and agreed that she was suffering from trigeminal neuralgia. He ordered imaging studies to rule out other causes and started her on anti-seizure medication for the pain.

Trigeminal neuralgia (also known as *tic douloureux*) is a sudden, excruciating burst of pain in the distribution of the trigeminal nerve, which supplies sensation to the entire face and mouth. The attacks are so severe that people are immobilized. Often there are *trigger zones*, discrete areas of the face or mouth, that when stimulated even by light touch, result in an attack of pain.

The typical pain that occurs in trigeminal neuralgia is intense, sharp, and usually lasts seconds, but can last as long as two minutes. These attacks are often called *lancinating*, meaning severe darting or stabbing pain. Many people equate the pain to an electrical shock. A *refractory*

The typical pain that occurs in trigeminal neuralgia is intense, sharp, and usually lasts seconds, but can last as long as two minutes.

period occurs after each attack. This is a portion of time when the next attack cannot be triggered. Trigeminal neuralgia can include periods of remission, during which the pain disappears for months to years at a time and then returns. Not all attacks have to be provoked by stimulating one of the trigger zones; many attacks occur spontaneously and, for that reason, people with trigeminal neuralgia often live in fear of their next attack.

The cause of trigeminal neuralgia is not fully understood. However, medical science believes it is caused by a loss of the protective outer layer of the trigeminal nerve (the *myelin sheath*). This may occur because an artery or vein rubs against the nerve near the place where the trigeminal nerve exits the skull. This is known as *vascular compression*. Some diseases (multiple sclerosis, for example) cause the loss of this protective layer, and a small percentage of these people also develop trigeminal neuralgia. Many of the surgical procedures that are performed are based on this belief and are aimed at either guarding the nerve from the blood vessels or at impairing the functioning of the nerve to decrease its activity.

Carbemazepine (Tegretol®) is an anticonvulsant medication that has been the treatment of choice for trigeminal neuralgia for many years. Trigeminal neuralgia is easily controlled in some people with medications and, recently, many new anticonvulsants have been developed, each of which has the potential to benefit people who suffer from this dreadful disorder. Others have initial success that dwindles with time, and still others have only limited success. For the latter two groups, surgical procedures are an option.

Diagnosing trigeminal neuralgia and other painful conditions is based on the headache sufferer's clinical presentation. There are no lab tests or imaging procedures that can confirm the diagnosis. The history the patient gives will lead the doctor to the correct diagnosis. On average, people who have facial pain will see 4 to 5 doctors before being referred to a pain clinic or specialist. To complicate matters, a wide range of facial pain syndromes exist, many of which have overlapping fea-

> The history the patient gives will lead the doctor to the correct diagnosis.

tures. Only by educating healthcare providers will more accurate and timely diagnosis of this disorder be accomplished.

Mr. White is a 40-year-old man who was kicked in the left side of his face by a horse one year ago when he was working on a horse farm. He lost consciousness and was taken to the local hospital, where he was treated surgically. He had two surgeries in the first three days to repair multiple facial fractures. His left orbit (the bones that support his left eye) was rebuilt. Luckily, Mr. White did not lose sight, but the left side of his face was numb after the swelling subsided, and his left eye was not as well supported as the right. His surgeons tried to repair the nerves, but immediately after the surgery, Mr. White had facial pain that radiated into his left upper teeth. The pain occasionally became more intense for a few days at a time, requiring him to seek seclusion and wait for the pain to subside.

After a year, Mr. White decided to seek further treatment. He had a continuous, aching pain in his left upper teeth that got worse when he tried to chew, and numbness in his left mid-face region. His pain got worse for two days, two to three times a month. Mr. White was sensitive to light, and the pain became pulsating during these exacerbations.

Mr. White was diagnosed with atypical facial pain, caused by a dysfunction of the sensory nerves in that region (also known as a neuropathy). The examination showed his teeth to be very sensitive when tapped, but the X-rays were normal. His face had a 50 percent loss of sensation to light touch on the left side. Mr. White was otherwise very healthy and appeared physically normal.

Mr. White was treated with amitriptyline (an antidepressant medication used for nerve pain), and within one month, he was virtually pain-free. With continued therapy, Mr. White is able to chew without sensitivity, his face has regained sensation, and his pain exacerbations are much less severe and less frequent.

The phrase *atypical facial pain* has been used since 1924 for pain in the facial region that does not fit the criteria for trigeminal neuralgia (see Table 16-1).

> The phrase *atypical facial pain* has been used since 1924 for pain in the facial region that does not fit the criteria for trigeminal neuralgia.

TABLE 16-1 Names Sometimes Given in Place of *Atypical Facial Pain*

• Stomatodynia	• Trigeminal nerve disorder
• Atypical odontalgia	• Trigeminal neuropathy
• Phantom tooth pain	• Trigeminal neuropathic pain
• Myogenic pain	• Oral and facial dysesthesias
• Traumatic neuralgia	

There is no uniform definition for atypical facial pain, and there is skeptical acceptance of this diagnosis among doctors and their patients, probably because of the variety of terms and the lack of understanding of what causes the pain. Basic scientific pain research is expanding the knowledge of how pain is transmitted by the nervous system, and this will allow doctors to better understand and treat these conditions. Pain research, new medication options, and increased clinical interest in the treatment of pain conditions have led to many new ideas and descriptions of the conditions that produce facial pain. Some day the diagnosis *atypical facial pain* will be replaced with many more precise diagnoses that we will better understand and be able to treat.

Ms. Smith is a 19-year-old college student who had a history of her jaw joint clicking whenever she opened her mouth. The clicking had been present for two years. It had never been painful and never resulted in any problems in chewing or talking. Ms. Smith recently went off to college and, during a game of basket-

ball, was bumped in the jaw. The next morning, she woke up and was unable to open her jaw. The clicking noises were gone and it was painful to open her mouth more than an inch.

Ms. Smith presented for an evaluation and was diagnosed as having an anterior displacement of the articular disc *in her left temporomandibular joint. In other words, the cartilage disc in the joint had slipped forward and was preventing her from opening her mouth normally. Every time she tried to open it, she stretched the tissues, which were full of blood vessels and nerves, causing pain. The joint itself was also sore from the trauma it had received during the game.*

Ms. Smith was treated with anti-inflammatory medications, instructed to rest for one week, and then physical therapy and an oral nightguard were to be used. Her symptoms subsided and her jaw was unlocked with the physical therapy exercises. Her jaw returned to its "normal" clicking after six weeks.

Ms. Smith's diagnosis is temporomandibular disorder, or TMD. *Temporomandibular disorder* is a collective phrase similar to *atypical facial pain*, within which there are multiple, more specific categories. Generally, TMDs can be split into two major groups: (1) those disorders involving the joint, and (2) those disorders involving the muscles used for chewing. The joint-related disorders include problems with the disc in the joint, arthritis of the joint, and trauma, tumors, and congenital malformations of the joint. The muscular disorders involve spasm, muscle fatigue, regional muscle pain (also known as *myofascial* pain), infections, and trauma to the muscles. There are several categories that fall under the heading of TMD and there are equally as many treatments, so treatment is individualized according to the findings on evaluation.

It is important for the headache sufferer to actively participate in the diagnosis and treatment, and to question the diagnosis when treatment is not working. Often, in very difficult cases, a multidisciplinary approach to therapy is recommended. This means that many specialties, including dentistry, neurology, endodontics, physical therapy, and psychology or psychiatry may be used in a team approach.

As stated earlier, people with facial pain frequently consult multiple doctors from many specialties before being given an appropriate diagno-

> It is important for the headache sufferer to actively participate in the diagnosis and treatment, and to question the diagnosis when treatment is not working.

sis and a course of treatment that affects their pain. These multiple doctor visits, referrals, and treatments are not only frustrating for the person who is in pain, but they are also quite costly. The face, head, and neck are treated by many doctors and, unfortunately, TMJ or TMD has become the generalized label for different pain syndromes that are now being better understood through research, and diagnosed more quickly by educated doctors.

Resources

AMERICAN COUNCIL FOR HEADACHE EDUCATION (ACHE)

19 Mantua Road
Mt. Royal, NJ 08061
Tel: 856-423-0258 800-255-ACHE (255-2243)
Fax: 856-423-0082
achehq@talley.com
http://www.achenet.org

ACHE is a nonprofit patient-health professional partnership dedicated to advancing the treatment and management of headache and to raising the public awareness of headache as a valid, biologically based illness. Its goals are to empower headache sufferers through education, and to support them by educating their families, employers, and the public in general.

ACHE was created in 1990 through an initiative of the American Headache Society (see below). Its website has extensive resource information a listing of support groups, and much more.

AMERICAN HEADACHE SOCIETY

19 Mantua Road
Mt. Royal, NJ 08061
Tel: 856-423-0043
Fax: 856-423-0082
ahshq@talley.com
http://www.ahsnet.org

The American Headache Society (AHS) is an organization of more than 2,400 physicians, health professionals and research scientists. Its website contains information primarily of interest to clinical professionals; this organization works closely with ACHE to produce educational programs and materials, coordinate its support groups, and undertake public awareness initiatives.

National Headache Foundation

820 N. Orleans
Suite 217
Chicago, IL 60610-3132
Tel: 773-388-6399 888-NHF-5552 (643-5552)
Fax: 773-525-7357
info@headaches.org
http://www.headaches.org

The Foundation's goals are: to serve as an information resource to headache sufferers, their families and the healthcare providers who treat them; to raise public awareness that headaches are a legitimate biological disease and sufferers should receive understanding and continuity of care; and to promote research into potential headache causes and treatments.

The Foundation website offers information on a variety of topics related to headache, information on support groups, information about clinical trials, publications, and much more.

TheBrainMatters

American Academy of Neurology Foundation
1080 Montreal Avenue
Saint Paul, MN 55116
www.thebrainmatters.org

This excellent educational resource provides information on a variety of topics related to migraine and other neurologic disorders. It is the patient education site of the American Academy of Neurology Foundation.

American Academy of Neurology

1080 Montreal Avenue
Saint Paul, MN 55116
www.aan.com

The AAN is the world's leading organization of neurology professionals and a strong advocate of public education, as reflected by its affiliated site, www.thebrainmatters.org. The AAN site itself is primarily for its physician members.

National Institute of Neurological Diseases and Stroke (NINDS)

National Institutes of Health
Bethesda, MD
http://www.ninds.nih.gov/

This site contains information of interest to people with a wide range of neurologic disorders, including migraine and other headaches.

Index

Note: Boldface numbers indicate illustrations.

causes of headache *(continued)*
  primary headache in, 32–34
  secondary headache and, 33, 34
  trigger vs., 19–21, **20**
  triggers vs. causes, 26
  types of headaches and, 21–23
Celebrex (*See* celecoxib)
celecoxib (Celebrex), 139
Celsius, 12
central scotoma, 14
cervical manipulation, 111
cervical pillow vs. neck disorders, 160
cervical spondylosis neck disorders, 158
cervicogenic headache (*See also* neck disorders), 155
chiropractic, 112
chlorpromazine (Thorazine), 91
chocolate, 72, 81
chronic tension headache, 124
chronic (transformed) migraine, 81–85
chronic daily headache, 137–138
citrus fruits, 81
clammy skin, 77
classic migraine, 62
classification of primary headache, 21, 22–23
Claviceps purpurea, 16
cluster headache, 6, 21, 22–23, 30, 129–135
  abortive treatment for, 135
  acute therapy for, 134–135
  aggravating and relieving factors for, 25–26
  associated symptoms with pain, 25–27
  behavior during headache and, 26–27
  causes of, 130–132, **131**
  chronic, 130
  frequency and timing of attacks and, 24–25
  gender and, 129
  genetic predisposition to headache, 27
  hypothalamus and, 130
  location and duration of pain in, 23–24
  maintenance therapy for, 133–134
  occipital nerve blocks in, 134
  oxygen therapy for, 134–135
  pain location in, 129–130, **131**
  pain severity and quality in, 25–27

cluster headache *(continued)*
  parasympathetic system and, 131
  preventive medication for, 133
  "suicide headache," 132
  surgical treatment of, 134
  sympathetic nervous system and, 131
  symptoms of, 129
  transitional treatment of, 134
  treatment of, 132–135
  trigeminal nerve and, 131
codeine, 90
coenzyme Q, 106–107
cognitive changes, 77, 79, 164, 165
cognitive-behavioral therapy, 128
coital headaches, 141
cold therapy, 111, 126
color distortion, 65
common migraine, 62
communicating with your doctor, 45, 48–49
  finding a good doctor for, 55–56
  skeptical doctors and, 55
Compazine (*See* prochlorperazine)
complete blood count (CBC), 30
complete migraine, 72
computed axial tomography (CT), 30–31, 40
  neck disorders, 160
  sinus headache and, 151
consciousness, alterations in, 65, 79
coordination (*See* walking and coordination problems)
Corgard (*See* nadolol)
corticosteroids, 92, 134, 154
coughing as trigger, 81
COX2 inhibitors, 139
craniocervical dystonia (CCD), 159, **159**
craniosacral therapy, 112
craniovertebral junction in neck disorders, 157
crepitus and neck disorders, 156
critical information for headache sufferers, 46
curing chronic headaches vs. management of, 48
cutaneous allodynia, 95

daily headache, 137–138
  hemicrania continua, 137–139
  new, persistent, 139–140

medication for treating migraines and
headaches *(continued)*
merperidine (Demerol), 90
methysergide (Sansert), 100–101
metoclopramide (Reglan), 91
metoprolol (Toprol), 98
mini-prophylaxis, 96, 102
morphine, 90
nadolol (Corgard), 98
naproxen sodium, 90
naratriptan (Amerge), 93–95
neuroleptic, 91–92
neuromodulating, 100
neurotoxic, 101–102
nonopioid, 90
nonsteroidal antiinflammatories
(NSAIDs) in, 89–91
nortriptyline (Pamelor), 99
ondansetron (Zofran), 91
opioid, 90–91, 103
oxycodone (Percocet; Lorcet), 90
prednisone, 92
preventive, 51, 64, 96–102
prochlorperazine (Compazine), 91
promethazine (Phenergan), 91
propoxyphene (Darvon), 90
propranolol (Inderal), 98
protriptyline (Vivactil), 99
rebound effect and (*See* rebound
headaches)
reducing dependence on, 47
rizatriptan (Maxalt), 93–95
selective serotonin and norepinephrine reuptake inhibitors (SNRIs),
99
selective serotonin reuptake
inhibitors (SSRIs), 99
sequential care and, 89
serotonin antagonist, 100–101
side effects of, 47–48
steroids, 92
stratified care and, 89
sumatriptan, 93–95
timolol (Blocadren), 98
topiramate (Topamax), 100
tricyclic antidepressants (TCAs), 99
triptan, 93–95
vasodilator, 98
verapamil (Calan), 99
zolmitriptan (Zomig), 93–95
Medieval treatments of headache,
12–13

meditation, 51, 114, 115–116
Medrol, 134
*Megrim, Sickheadache, and Some Allied
Disorders,* 13
meninges inflammation and
migraine, 70
meningitis, 28, 32, 34, 39–40
menopause, 27, 63–64, 80
menstrual cycle and migraine, 26, 33,
63–64, 79–81, 96, 102
meperidine (Demerol), 90
meridians, in acupressure/acupuncture
treatment, 111
methysergide (Sansert), 100–101
metoclopramide (Reglan), 91
metoprolol (Toprol), 98
Midrin (*See* butalbital)
migraine, 30, 33, 34, 61–85
acute, 87–89
age of onset for, 71–72, **71**
aggravating and relieving factors for,
25–26
allodynia and, 70, 71, 77, 95
associated symptoms with pain,
25–27
aura and, 64–65, 67–68, 73
auraless, 62–64
basilar, 65, 78–79
behavior during headache and,
26–27
Bickerstaff Syndrome and, 65
brain areas generating, 68–70, **70**
brain wave activity during, 67–68,
68, 69
brain wave hyperexcitability/hyper-
sensitivity in, 67
causes of, 61–70
chronic (transformed), 81–85
analgesic overuse and, 82–85
early chronic daily headache as, 82
prevalence of, 82
rebound headache and, 82–85
classic, 62
classification and definition of,
61–62
common, 62
complete, 72
early vs. late medical treatment of,
95–96
equivalents to, 79
frequency and timing of attacks and,
24–25

neck disorders *(continued)*
  developmental anomalies and abnor-
    malities in, 157
  dystonia and, 159
  magnetic resonance imaging (MRI)
    and, 160
  medication to treat, 160–161
  multiple myeloma and, 157
  nerve blocks in, 160–161
  occiput pain in, 156, 157
  osteomyelitis and, 157
  subocciptal pain in, 157
  trauma and, 157, 158
  treatment of, 160
  x-rays and, 160
nerve blocks
  cluster headache and, 134
  neck disorders, 160–161
nerve storms, 13, 23–24, 66
neurogenic inflammation theory of
  migraine, 66
neuroleptics, 91–92
neurologic examination, 28–32
neurologists, 5
neurology, 13
neuromodulating medications, 100
Neurotonin *(See* gabapentin)
neurotoxic medications, 101–102
neurotransmitters *(See also* serotonin),
  66
neurovascular theory of migraine, 66
new daily persistent headache,
  139–140
nineteenth century treatment of
  headache, 13–15
nitrates, 81
nitroglycerin headaches, 26
No–Doz *(See* caffeine)
noise *(See* sound sensitivity)
nonopioid medications, 90
nonprescription *(See also* over the
  counter) medication, 4, 27, 83
nonsteroidal antiinflammatories
  (NSAIDs), 83, 89–91, 96, 125,
  138–139, 160
nortriptyline (Pamelor), 99
nose/sinus disease *(See* sinus headache
  and nasal disease)
Novocaine, 153
numbers of people suffering migraine,
  in U.S., 7, 70–72
numbness and tingling, 5, 42, 74, **74**

occipital nerve blocks in cluster
  headache, 134
occiput pain in neck disorders, 156,
  157
odor sensitivity, 21, 63, 74
ondansetron (Zofran), 91
opioid medications, 90–91, 103, 135
opium, 12
orthostatic hypotension, 98
osteomyelitis and neck disorders, 157
ostiomeatal complex,, 150, **150**
Othello and traditional headache
  treatment, 12–13
over the counter (OTC), ix
oxycodone (Percocet; Lorcet), 84, 90,
  103

pain severity and quality in, 25–27,
  76–77
pallor, 77
Pamelor *(See* nortriptyline), 99
papilledema, 28–29
parasympathetic system, cluster
  headache and, 131
paroxysmal hemicrania, 137
passionflower, 109
past history of headache, 27
patient education, ix
  American Council for Headache
    Education (ACHE) support
    groups, 177–179
peppermint oil, 108
Percocet *(See* oxycodone), 90
Personal Memoirs of Ulysses S. Grant, , 15
personality and migraine, 15
Petadolex *(See* butterbur root)
Peters, 17
Phenergan *(See* promethazine)
phonophobia *(See* sound sensitivity)
phosphenes *(See also* flashing lights),
  77
physical and neurologic examination,
  28–32, 46
  computed tomography (CT) in,
    30–31
  diagnostic testing in, 29, 33, 29
  electroencephalograph (EEG) in, 30
  lumbar puncture in, 31–32, **32**
  magnetic resonance angiography in,
    31
  magnetic resonance imaging (MRI)
    in, 30–31

weakness, 40, 42, 74
weather as trigger, 51, 81
weekend headache, 80–81
West Nile virus, 40
whiplash (*See* trauma and neck
    disorders)
willow tree extract (*Salix alba*), 108
wine, 21, 26, 81
Wolff, Harold, 15

x-rays and neck disorders, 160

yawning, 73
yoga, 51, 113

Zofran (*See* ondansetron)
zolmitriptan (Zomig), 93–95
Zomig (*See* zolmitriptan)
zone therapy (reflexology), 113